PENGUIN BOOKS

LIVING WITH ENERGY

Ronald Alves was raised on a diversified farm in central California and, after completing his college studies, went on to teach vocational agriculture on the high-school level for four years. Disillusioned with what was happening in the United States in the late 1960s, he sought a far-away place from which he could view the situation objectively. He chose the Orient and while there evolved an alternative way of seeing, a viewpoint that was to be solidified during his graduate work in Social Ecology at Goddard College, Vermont. Alves is currently teaching in the Agriculture Department at Modesto Junior College; operating a small farm with his wife, Bernie, and son, Jason; and deeply involved in programs and projects concerning ecological agriculture, aquaculture, and integrated systems.

Born in Los Angeles in 1942, the year the local spinach crop failed because of smog, Charles Milligan was presented with his first Minolta while a sophomore at the Chouinard Art Institute. He has been in and out of corporate art directorships for twelve years. While contesting the construction of a nuclear power plant in Modesto, where he now lives with his wife, Estelle, a social worker and incipient poet, he searched in vain for a book just like *Living with Energy*. Convinced that there was not one to be found, he and Alves decided to fill this apparent gap. At present, Milligan is working on related and unrelated photo essays and a large sculptured organic garden.

Ralph Nader's name has become synonymous with the fight for justice. Through his organization, the Center for Study of Responsive Law, he and his "raiders" conduct research into the possible abuse of public interest by business and governmental groups. His concern with the energy situation and its future will, it is hoped, prompt the enactment of appropriate legislation.

Living with Energy

Text by **Ronald Alves**
Photographs by **Charles Milligan**
Preface by **Ralph Nader**

PENGUIN BOOKS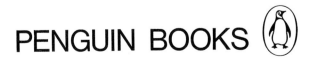

Penguin Books Ltd, Harmondsworth,
Middlesex, England
Penguin Books, 625 Madison Avenue,
New York, New York 10022 U.S.A.
Penguin Books Australia Ltd, Ringwood,
Victoria, Australia
Penguin Books Canada Limited, 2801 John Street,
Markham, Ontario, Canada L3R 1B4
Penguin Books (N.Z.) Ltd, 182–190 Wairau Road,
Auckland 10, New Zealand

First published in the United States of America
in simultaneous hardcover and paperback editions
by The Viking Press and Penguin Books 1978

Library of Congress Cataloging in Publication Data
Alves, Ronald, 1942—
Living with energy.
Bibliography: p.
1. Power resources. 2. Energy conservation.
I. Milligan, Charles, 1942—   II. Title.
[TJ163.2.A47   1977]   333.7   77–9049
ISBN 0 14 00.4681 X

Printed in Japan by Dai Nippon
Printing Co., Tokyo
Set in Linotype Helvetica

Acknowledgments
   A few special individuals and groups
contributed to this book above and beyond what
was asked of them. Some served as motivators
and others gave us physical assistance; we are
especially indebted to the following: *Nancy
Nickum Bailey, John Brand, Gary DeLoss,
Ecology Action Educational Institute of Modesto,
John Hammond, Malcolm Lillywhite, Fran and
Stan Milic, Modesto Peace Life Center, Nels
Overgaard, Pacific Gas and Electric, Rob Quigley,
Richard Schuettge, Social Ecology Program at
Goddard College, Kathleen Spencer, Florence
van Dresser,* and *Frank Verprauskus.*
   Our thanks also go to the hundreds of people
who have shared "their place to throw a sleeping
bag" with us. Some are included in the pages to
follow, but many are not. It is all of these people,
the "doers," who are the real authors of *Living
with Energy.*

To Estelle and Bernie

Contents

Preface

Giant energy companies and electric utilities promote the use of expensive energy technologies dependent on the fossil fuels and uranium they control. They make large profits from managing investments in such high technologies. Thus they promote the practice of heating homes to temperatures in the seventies with electricity generated by atomic power plants with reactor core temperatures of thousands of degrees. This use of high technology may increase the profits of investors in electric utilities and atomic power, but it is technologically and thermodynamically as appropriate as cutting butter with a chainsaw.

The alternative energy pioneers described in this book prefer the common-sense approach of cutting butter with a butter knife. They are committed to satisfying their energy needs with safe and environmentally benign *appropriate* technologies such as better building design, solar heating, and wind power. Rather than invent new technologies, these pioneers are substituting existing but largely unused appropriate technologies for wasteful high technologies.

Some of the technologies discussed in this book are ancient. Reliance on these alternative energy sources, however, does not foreclose technological innovation. Indeed, appropriate technologies lend themselves to individual experimentation and improvement. Thus alternative energy pioneers often make novel refinements of building design concepts and natural energy systems that have been understood and used in one fashion or another for thousands of years.

Widespread adoption of these modern examples of energy conservation and use of renewable energy sources would reduce our reliance on fossil fuels and atomic power. Our society's energy efficiency, economic well-being, environmental quality, and national security would be improved. A high priority on the citizen action agenda should be the recognition of these massive, realizable benefits that encourage a shift in public policies from high technologies to appropriate technologies in order to meet our energy needs.

—Ralph Nader

6

Introduction

We have tried to capture real people in a fashion that describes them at their best—living within the constraints of their own creativity, ideas, and inventions. This is not a how-to book, but a blueprint of energy, architectural, and life-style alternatives. These alternatives, economically practical and readily available at the present time, are waiting to be used.

Contrary to general belief, alternative energy buffs are not reverting to a more primitive life-style. These energy pioneers are simply learning to live in greater harmony with the renewable resources at hand. A solar heating system is both practical and economical, and though an active system may not be economically justifiable in every situation, there are choices among the solar uses. In almost all cases passive heating and cooling systems (no pumps or other moving parts) are not too expensive. In fact, most of us fail to realize that with the inevitable increase in fossil-fuel prices, we can't afford not to have some energy-conserving application. The argument that the use of alternative energy is still a few years away just isn't true (the ancients used it rather successfully). Alternative energy devices will no doubt improve, but well-engineered alternative energy systems are available today.

There will be changes in our living patterns. The changes that we notice first will be those that remove some of our "necessary" modern conveniences. The acceptance of little inconveniences is not as important as restyling our attitudes—our levels of awareness. Perhaps the greatest single gesture any individual can make is to develop a genuine conservation consciousness. This certainly doesn't mean we must turn off lights and heat and huddle in the middle of a dingy room with an old army blanket draped around us. We will not have to relinquish our total life-style (which has many good points) but we will have to establish criteria for living a gentler life. The template for this life has been molded. We now need to educate ourselves to implement it on a grass-roots level.

The people referred to in *Living with Energy* are a cross section of the pioneers who are carrying out the initial educational process. Through their experiences, these people will enable us to temper the transition from a fossil-fuel/nuclear-based existence to a more steady-state, conservation-conscious vitality. Their homes, generators, and integrated systems are shown here to introduce the available alternatives. A comprehensive regional access section is also included for further exploration.

We hope *Living with Energy* will help you. If you find an idea here you can adapt to your own situation, we will feel we've accomplished one of our purposes. The time to act is now, because we are at a point where we are running out of stored energy sources and befouling the environment on all fronts. How will the dilemma be resolved? How do we get from here to there, from the wanton theft of resources to integration in the network of nature? *Living with Energy* presents some options. A few individuals, one piece of legislation, an organization, a consciousness—any of these may not be very significant alone, but together they form the framework on which people can build to truly *live,* rather than exist, in the future.

House-Turned-Temple

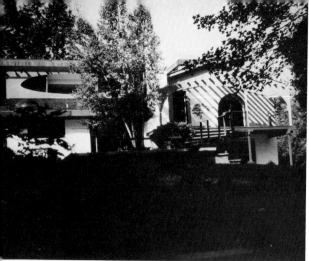

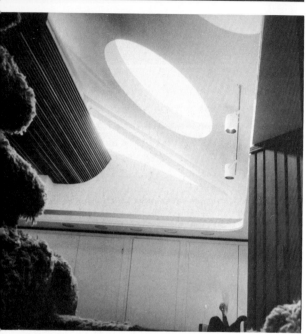

Al Zabrek, architect and resident of this house, describes it as a $50,000 home in a $100,000 neighborhood with a $200,000 look. In 1972 this conventional-looking brick-fronted Georgetown home was consumed by fire. From those ashes Al Zabrek helped to create a multifaceted, multiuse home. Though the house is more architecturally innovative than it is energy conserving, it incorporates a number of noteworthy conservation features.

Insulation is an important energy-saving aspect: 15 centimeters (6 inches) of fiberglass wreathe the entire structure. Closets, built between the insulated wall and the rooms they serve, are air-lock buffer zones between the heated rooms and the cold outside. Special attention has been paid to lighting, and energy is conserved through the use of fluorescent lights and skylights. The domed skylights give the house a futuristic look and provide the means for a kinetic lighting drama throughout the day. A large oval window high on the eastern side of the house provides additional light and can be opened for venting purposes during the hot, sticky summers. The west windows are either shaded with an attractive array of arching slats or painted a quarter-bronze tone to deflect the hot afternoon sun.

When Zabrek had the house rebuilt, he did it with modularization in mind. Although there is a nice contiguous flow between the various spaces, many of them can be made into smaller modules.

For instance, by moving a couple of pieces of furniture and closing doors, Al was able to make a hallway into a conference room he calls the "Manhattan Project." Even from the outside, the house has many different faces. The front looks like a business office on one side and a typical Georgetown house on the other. (That Georgetown look probably makes this original home more acceptable to the neighbors.) The high ceiling and a set of double sliding glass doors open onto a tree-lined patio deck to give the house a townhouse-with-a-California-flair look. From this deck a delicate winding stairway leads up to a second-floor bedroom. The four split-level floors, the use of mirrors, and built-in modular furniture create the effect of a Hollywood set.

The bedroom is located at the highest elevation, a good idea because heat rises. The room—floors, walls, and ceiling—is com-

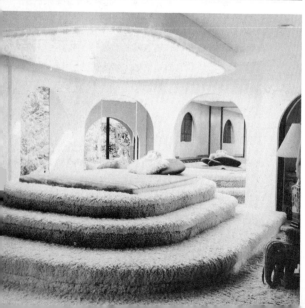

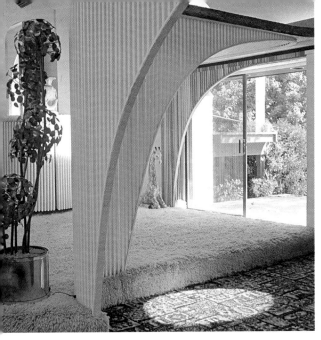

pletely carpeted, and mirrors cover much of the walls and ceiling. A sliding glass door leads to a Japanese patio, and a Romeo-and-Juliet windowed balcony is there for early-morning musing. The water bed is at the top of a three-tiered terrace, and a control panel for adjusting lights, operating the stereo system, and raising and lowering a mirrored skylight, is recessed next to the bed. The highlight of an evening's activities, at least for the more athletic, might be diving through the skylight onto the water bed below.

Al describes this house-turned-temple as the house of the future. He feels that buildings such as his give architects the initiative to really make use of their talents. A home can be a work of art that is visually acceptable, protects against excessive loss of energy, and furnishes the inhabitants with the dynamic experience necessary for a healthy state of mind.

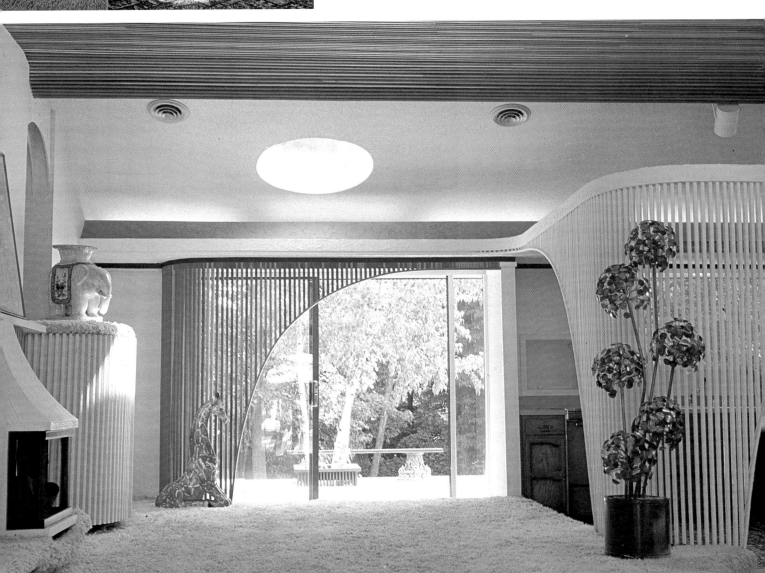

A Fantasy of Foam

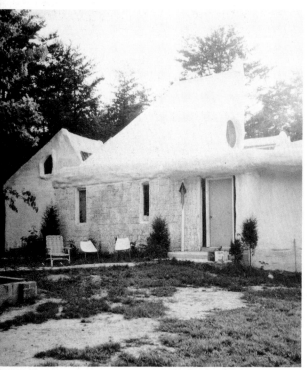

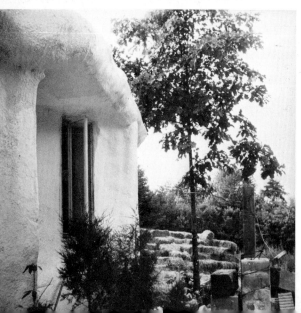

Hansel and Gretel might like to nibble on this fantastic house. More than likely, however, one would mistake this structure for a piece of architecture from the twenty-first century. But this house of curves, bulges, and sweeping lines is a very real 1970s home, constructed of a wood and plywood frame that has been sprayed with urethane foam. Why would anyone construct such a building?

Of the many energy-conservation alternatives, the use of insulation is probably the most cost effective. A logical approach to the use of insulation would be to construct a home from the insulation itself—which is exactly what the Thomas Lindseys of eastern Virginia have done.

Urethane foam, which has about twice the insulating value of fiberglass, is a cellular structure made when gas is blown through a plastic resin material. For the Lindsey home, the gasification of the urethane was performed as it was blown onto a framework. Usually, urethane is fire resistant, but if it is subjected to intense heat, poisonous cyanide gas can be released. Urethane also deteriorates in ultraviolet light. Both these problems can be overcome by the use of fireproof paint. Tom Lindsey had his house painted with Medusa cement, thereby changing it from an orange structure in conflict with the environment to a soft white building that snuggles in comfortably with the surrounding vegetation.

The Lindseys have chosen to combine conservation with creative design. For example, the use of an average thickness of 7.5 centimeters (3 inches) of urethane foam gives the house a resistance factor of 22. This insulation, coupled with the lack of any open joints (even the windows were foamed in), equals a very energy-conserving house. Tom Lindsey estimates that his electric baseboard heating costs will run about $600 per year, while his neighbors with homes of similar size and comparable heating systems, but without the benefit of insulation, will spend $1200. Polyfoam, sprayed on an assortment of forms, enables one to create exciting structures and interior spaces. Private spaces, furniture, and even rooftop patios can be foamed into place.

There is an excellent use of space in the house, for the foaming construction technique allows alcoves and cubicles to be added to central areas. The six bedrooms and a dressing room fit conveniently around a central bath–laundry space. Five of the bedrooms enter into a large playroom area. The whole sleeping complex, along with a family area and a work space, converge on a centrally located living room. Because the urethane technique lends itself to modularization, the basic components of a house and additional rooms can be easily built as family size increases or as more money becomes available.

Though polyfoam houses tend to maintain a high relative humidity, when inside temperatures go as low as 19° C. (66° F.) the occupants feel very comfortable. The more humid the air, the less moisture the body gives off; the less moisture lost, the warmer the person will feel. In the summertime the house may become uncomfortable, but opening a few windows will let in the cooler dry air from the outside. The stack effect directs warm air upward and out. Many shade trees further summer cooling.

Construction costs were about the same as for a conventional dwelling. At present, urethane foam may not be considered desirable by lending and building institutions, but we may see more foam houses in the future as they are proved fire-safe and we learn to appreciate the structural strength and longevity of this energy-conserving material.

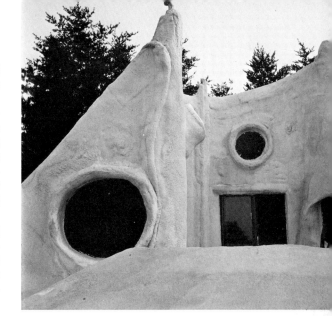

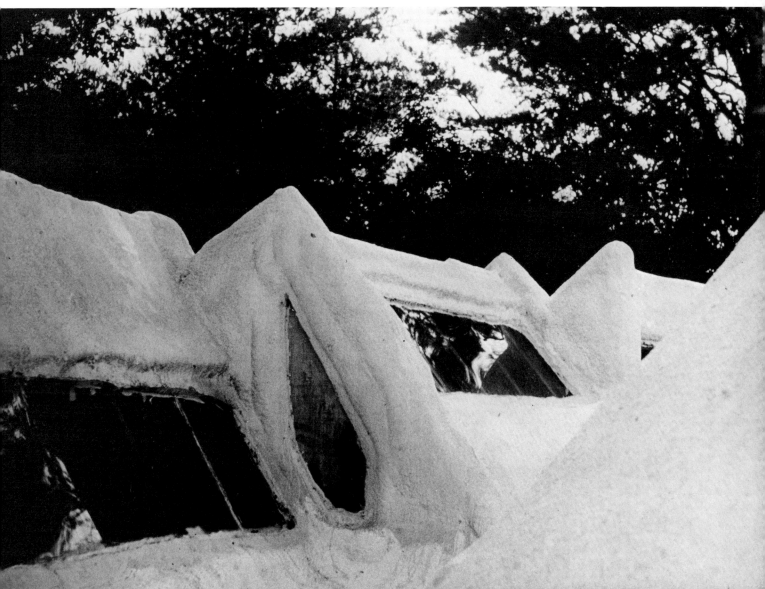

Bastida's Solarium Houses

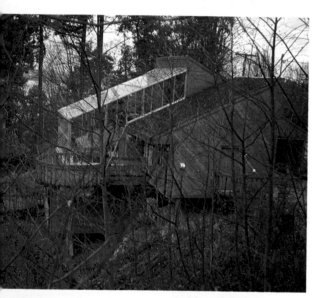

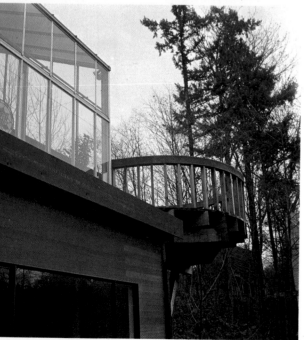

Fantasize about a house that is capable of reaching out and bringing in the outside. Imagine living in a place that changes with the seasons, daily, even hourly—so much so that it seems alive. Allow yourself the pleasure of experiencing a room that is so bright and cheery you don't want to leave. William Bastida's Mercer Island, Washington, home designs not only accomplish the above, but also save money by conserving energy.

Architect Bastida's passive solar design had to contend with a climate where rain falls on the average more than 150 days per year. The sun shines only 19 percent of the daylight hours in December and 49 percent of the time in July. But temperatures are mild and seldom average below 5° C. (41° F.) for any length of time. Houses in his native France, where the climate is similar, were designed with passive solar concepts and worked well. Why wouldn't they work in the Seattle area? It looks as though Bill Bastida is proving they will.

Fitting the site almost perfectly, this 186-square-meter (2000-square foot) solar home is internally divided into five split-levels and features a southern exposure through 37 square meters (400 square feet) of single-layered glass windows. To demonstrate the intricacy of site orientation, during the peak summer season the large conifers on the southwestern side of the house begin to shade the glassed area at about 2:30 p.m., yet they do not interfere with the sun in the wintertime. The vertical is conventional, allowing the winter sun to penetrate for gains in direct heating. The glass roof is reflective, enabling the summer sun to be reflected about 85 percent. This type of construction is about 5–10 percent more expensive than the average house, but it more than makes up for the additional expense in energy savings. Although the house has not been formally monitored, during the first winter after it was built the December heating cost for an electric baseboard system was $35. The owners of a nonsolarized house of similar size in the same area spent $176 for heating oil.

The house is oriented south for more than the purpose of sun-gathering. The street is on the north side, and by making the north wall solid (only a few windows were constructed), much street noise was screened out, as well as the cold winds from the Gulf of Alaska that pass over the house.

In addition, two interesting lighting concepts are employed. Task lighting, featuring mobile overhead lamps, reduces electricity

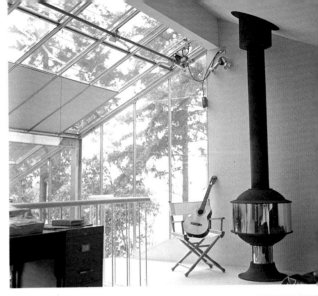

costs by enabling one to direct light only to where it is needed. The strip fluorescent lights are fronted by chrome reflectors that direct the light to the light-hued walls. This reflected light then bathes the entire area in soft, nonglaring illumination, giving one the sensation of warmth and radiance.

The location of the circular fireplace makes it more efficient than a conventional fireplace in the external wall. In addition, the chromed edges of the fireplace serve to reflect additional heat into the living space, rather than allowing it to pass upward to the rafters.

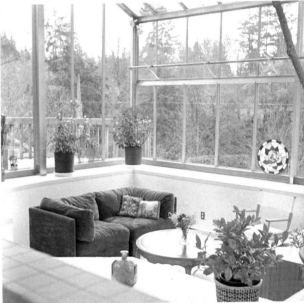

The backup heating system is a series of electric baseboard heaters. Mr. Bastida feels that these electric heaters, if properly placed near the windows, will heat more economically than oil-fired heaters. The warm air circulates away from the windows, rather than toward them. This minimizes energy needs, because less heat is lost through the glass. In tune with attempts to minimize energy consumption, each room is equipped with its own thermostat, so that the amount of heat in each room can be independently controlled.

William Bastida's architecture will play an important role in educating the Pacific Northwest to more energy-efficient housing. In addition to retrofitting homes, he has designed a veterinary hospital and his own home and office.

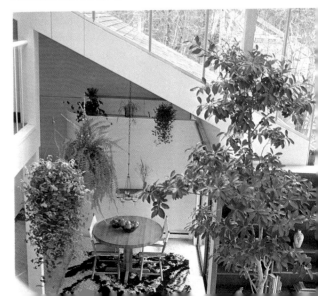

Another Brand of Solar Energy

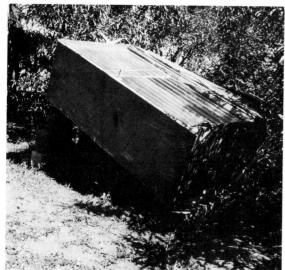

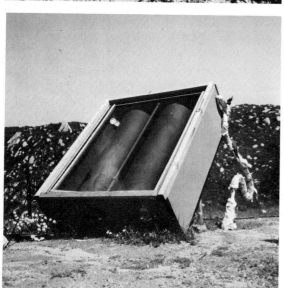

President of the Southern California Solar Energy Association, John Brand is a firm believer in "low-technology solar applications." He and his wife, Ildiko, are the major forces behind the SCSEA, which disseminates information, publishes a quarterly newsletter, and most important, educates people—including the organization's 300-plus membership—about the practical alternatives available to them.

At his San Diego home, John has used the sun in a number of ways: a solar water heater and a solar still were among his first ventures, and a second water heater was constructed from scrounged materials that cost only $20. This second heater supplies John and Ildiko with 90 percent of their yearly hot-water needs.

One of their neighbors, Larry Watson, benefited from an earlier Brand idea. John scrounged an old refrigerator, painted the inside black, and placed a black painted water tank in the box. He then covered the opening with two layers of transparent plastic, and the result was the most inexpensive solar hot-water heater money couldn't buy. The heater, installed in Larry's backyard, saves considerable money each month in electric water-heating bills and has paid for itself many times over.

The almost passive space heating and cooling system is truly unique. John was inspired by the ideas of Frenchman Eric Trombe, Steve Baer of Zomeworks, and the Kalwall Corporation of New Hampshire. John stacked ten water-filled 220-liter (55-gallon) barrels on the southwest wall of a 3 × 9 meter (10 × 30 foot) enclosed porch that was added to a 2.4 × 12 meter (8 × 40 foot) trailer house. The barrels are enclosed in this small area by a 6.5 square meter (70 square foot) sheet of transparent tedlar-coated fiberglass. Covering the fiberglass is an insulated wall that is hinged at the bottom and foil-coated on the inside. When this wall is lowered, the barrels are exposed to the sun, and the water in them is heated. The foil enhances the heating by reflecting more sun onto the barrels. After three days of continuous sun, the water in the barrels has reached a temperature of 160° F. At night John and Ildiko close the portable wall and start a small fan (the only active aspect of the heating system) to draw air across the barrels and blow it into the living space. With the fan at a ceiling-high vent in the barrel room and a vent to admit house air on the opposite side at floor level, there is a constant current of air blowing the barrel heat back into the house. In the summertime the opening of the portable

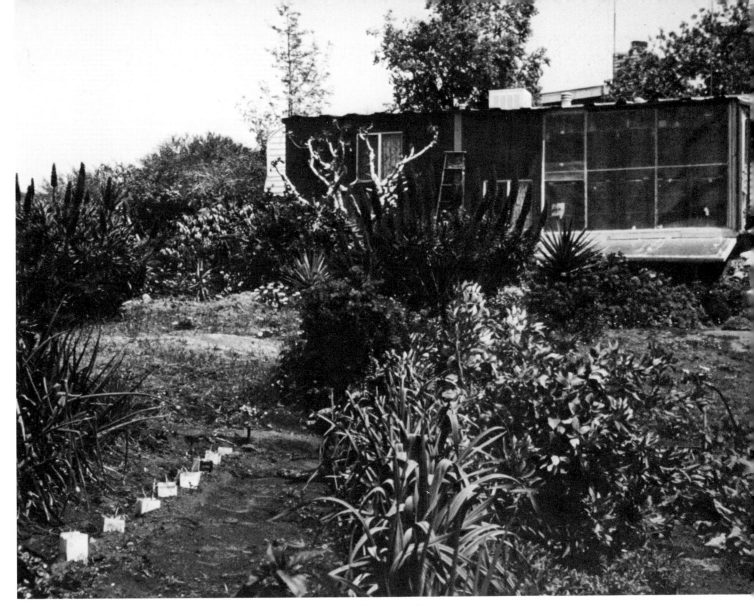

wall is done at night so the water barrels cool. During the day, air circulated across them results in cool air being blown into the house. The entire solar heater and air conditioner cost $75.

John Brand was a philosophy student while in college. This amazes people when they consider all of the creative ideas and designs in alternative energy that have emerged from his backyard. I asked John how he managed to produce all these practical devices with this limited background. John replied, "I've never been trained not to do what I can't do." Armed with such a philosophy, Brand-new ideas and creativity may well be the alternative technological breakthroughs that help keep our lives pleasant. Furthermore, John feels that in order to achieve saner energy-use standards, it is necessary to blend modern technology with the counterculture ideas. Through this balance we will more rapidly achieve living patterns within the margins of tolerance of the environment.

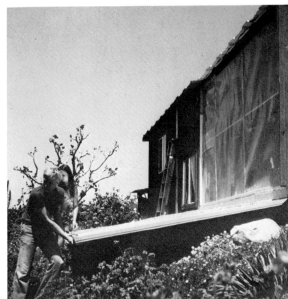

Water Beds in the Sky

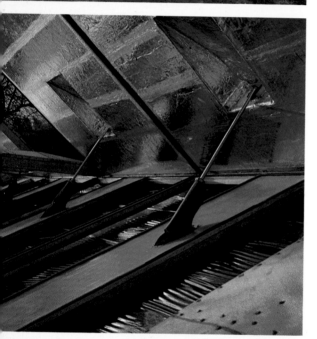

Imagine a house in the middle of California's hot central valley, without benefit of air conditioning and central heating, that has never been hotter than 25° C. (77° F.) or colder than 17° C. (63° F.) when the temperature outside registered —5° C. (23° F.). The house is designed to respond inversely to nature's climate— when it's hot outside the house is cool, and when it's cold outside the house is warm.

This environmentally conceived solar home has no collector panels, there are no pumps, and moving parts have been reduced to a near minimum. In fact, the elaborate hydraulic system used to raise and lower the insulated roof panels could just as easily be a manual crank.

Located on a knoll overlooking an almond orchard, this handsome house was designed by Jon Hammond at the request of a University of California professor who felt the need to conserve both energy and money. The house has fulfilled these criteria beautifully. To heat it, one-half cord of wood per year is burned, which means a $600 annual saving in heating costs. Each day one minute's worth of electricity is used in a small motor to raise and lower the insulated panels. This energy expenditure is the entire requirement for meeting heating and cooling needs! In addition, the house is cost competitive. Its 107 square meters (1150 square feet) cost approximately $25,000 in 1974–1975. Along with saving money, the owners have the pleasure of knowing that they are living in harmony with the environment.

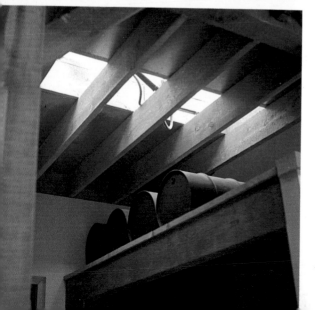

The house is filled with small devices to capture the sun's energy. Heat sinks radiate the captured solar energy back to the living space for warmth in the winter and to the outside atmosphere for coolth in the summer. Tastefully situated 220-liter (55-gallon) black painted drums are part of the interior decor. A cement floor, which has been brightened with throw rugs, soaks up a great deal of midday sun. The major source for heating and cooling is 7300 kilograms (16,000 pounds) of water in eight "water beds" on the roof. Just imagine the BTUs of energy that are captured when the temperature of this water is raised from 22° C. to 33°C. (72° F. to 92° F.) in a single day. When properly utilized, these beds temper the house's temperature fluctuations year-round. To minimize exchange with the outside atmosphere, the house is snugly insulated, and all windows have insulated panels or shutters covering them. All this is essential if the house is to work properly.

16

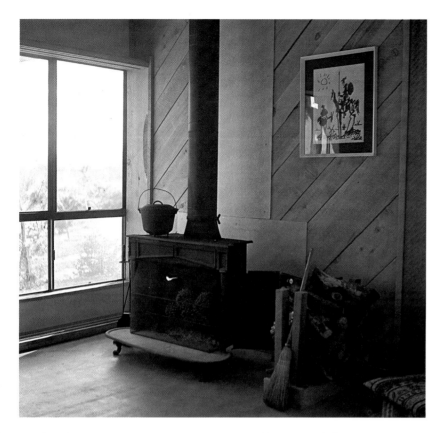

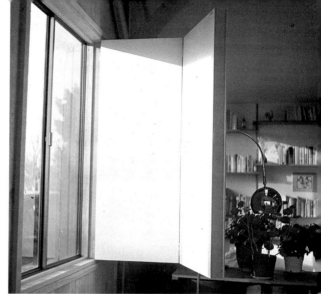

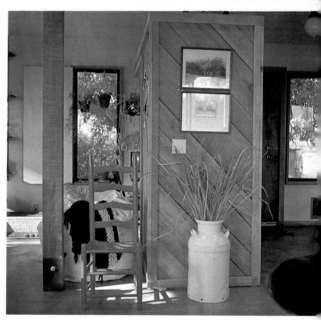

California's dry summer climate with day-night temperature differences of 22° C. to 28° C. (40° F. to 50° F.) makes this passive system ideal for cooling, too. During the daytime the insulated roof panels are closed. The water beds absorb the house heat created internally. The water is exposed to the cool night sky so that by the next day it too will be cooled sufficiently to remove heat from the house again. The day in which the house achieved its all-time high of 25°C. (77°F.), it was 42°C. (108°F.) outside. An electricity-guzzling air conditioner could do no better than this solar house.

Of course, there are times when the sun doesn't shine. Two Franklin stoves, one in the bedroom and one in the living room, provide all the necessary backup heat. Since this solar home was one of the first of its kind in the north central valley of California, the architect, builder, and owner were not sure that it was going to work. To protect the investment, a conventional natural-gas heater was included in the house. As of this writing, the pilot light on the heater has never been lit.

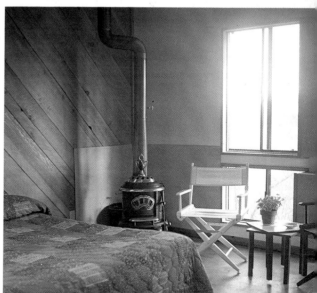

Living Systems, Inc.

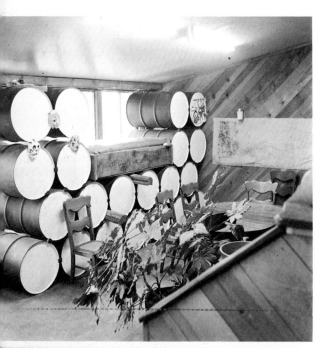

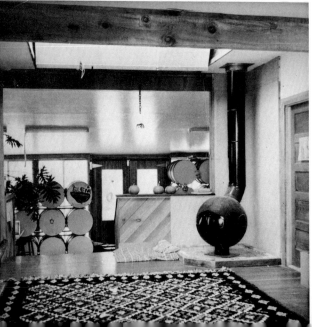

When walking into Jon and Lori Hammond's house, one is immediately confronted with dogs, kids, and a stack of 220-liter (55-gallon) drums painted black and white.

The Hammond house has been remodeled to take full advantage of the sun's energy, and the drums are the thermal sinks that radiate warmth in winter and coolness in summer.

Jon Hammond, writer, scientist, landscape and building architect, and consultant, is a pioneer in the development of integrated alternative energy systems. He and his family not only promote energy conservation, they live a life-style that exemplifies their beliefs, a life-style that is comfortable by any standards.

Most of the work in retrofitting (remodeling) this vintage farmhouse was done by Jon and Lori. Before any solar devices were incorporated, they insulated the house as well as they could because they knew that without proper insulation, solarizing would be inconsequential. A concrete floor in the kitchen and one in the dining room (located in the southern wing exposure) were added.

Their energy system is based on the "drum-wall" theme. The south wall is comprised of a stack of 220-liter (55-gallon) black painted drums that are filled with water and fronted entirely with glass. They, and the concrete floor, are heated by the sun during winter days and relinquish that heat to the living space after the sun goes down. Insulated panels cover the south-facing glass, preventing undue evening heat loss from the sun-warmed barrels and floor. The grapevine snaking its way across the trellis above and to the south of the barreled wall does not impede winter sun and provides cooling shade for the whole patio in the summer.

Insulated shutters cover windows that were designed for specific reasons: one small north-facing window looks onto a bird's nest, another enables one to watch the children while doing work in the kitchen. The bright and colorful interior of the house is bathed in natural light from a skylight. The living room and Jon's research shop each have a recycled marker buoy that has been cleverly disguised as a wood stove—a good idea of how to make something useful out of a former throwaway.

To further integrate energy conservation into their home, the Hammonds have installed a thermosiphon solar water heater. The sun-heated water moves from the collector panel via convection currents into a 360-liter (90-gallon) storage tank in the attic. This solar-heated water is backed up by a conventional hot-water heater—natural gas is used to heat water only when the sun can't do the entire job, which is less than 30 percent of the time.

Jon is the founder of Living Systems, Inc., an organization that designs private and public alternative energy buildings and engages in political activities to encourage the enactment of new guidelines promoting energy conservation. Living Systems' physical plant is a combination workshop, office, and research laboratory. The headquarters building has been structured to reduce energy consumption. Its 60-degree south-facing windows capture the maximum amount of energy from the winter sun. The interior is heavily insulated, and a dirt berm covers all but the entrances. The overhang on the south windows shades out most of the summer sun, but allows more to enter the building in the fall and winter.

In addition to its designs, Living Systems also researches specific ways and means to conserve energy. A row of concrete blocks is carefully monitored by a continuous printout to determine which type will make the most economic heat-lag wall. An alternating black and white roofing bank is being tested for the city of Sacramento to determine the efficiency of different rooftop colors. In this case, Jon and company are looking at maximum and minimum solar absorptiveness and reflectivity. The colorful pipe culverts will become part of a wall called a solar battery because it will absorb and store heat energy in a new state building in Sacramento. Living Systems is the organization carrying out the design for this passively oriented state office building.

The aim of Living Systems can be summed up in this paraphrased statement from Jon Hammond's proposal for an Energy Conservation Service: If we are to continue to compete in the world we must improve our energy efficiency. The most practical way to do this is through energy conservation. The numerous small increments of energy that can be conserved will add up to large savings. This conservation need can be met only if we recognize our situation and are willing to commit a large portion of our creativity and capital to the task. It is cheaper to save energy than to generate new energy.

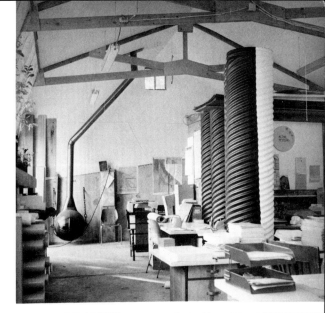

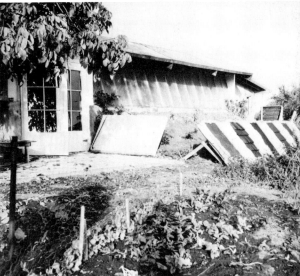

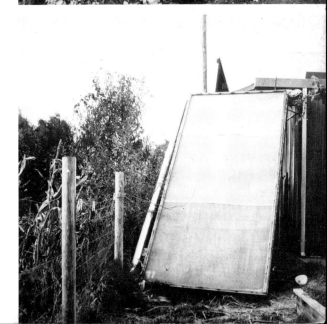

19

The Kelbaughs' Trombe Adventure

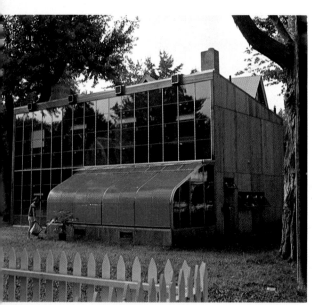

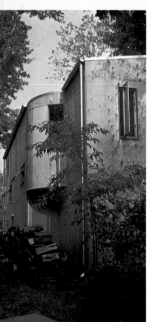

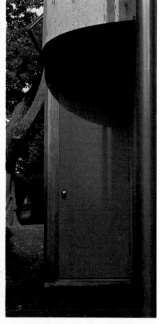

France has developed a number of notable alternative energy applications, including several wind generators, like the Aerowatt, and a large solar furnace, located at the Solar Energy Laboratory at Odeillo. The furnace deserves special mention because of its size—61 meters (200 feet)—and performance—temperatures up to 3315° C. (6000° F.)—but France's most significant contribution to the use of renewable energy resources in the home is the Trombe wall.

Invented by French solar energy pioneer Dr. Felix Trombe, this home construction technique is a most successful passive means of heating a room or an entire building. (See also the Total Environmental Action house, page 26.)

Doug Kelbaugh, an architect and solar engineer, and his wife modified the basic Trombe design with the addition of a greenhouse and basement in building their 195-square-meter (2100-square-foot) home. The two-story structure satisfies the occupants' needs and the neighborhood's requirements.

The focus around which the entire house was planned is a massive 38-centimeter (15-inch) concrete wall, which became the house's south wall and acts as a thermal sink. The Trombe wall, broken through for upstairs and downstairs windows at critical points, is painted with Nextal, a black selective absorptive coating. Two layers of glass, 2.5 centimeters (1 inch) apart and 15 centimeters (6 inches) from the concrete, cover the exterior south wall. Vents at the top and bottom of the concrete wall are necessary for transferring heat, and it is important that the upper vent be twice as large as the lower. The vents themselves should total about one-half the cross-sectional area of the area they serve.

The Trombe wall acts like the heat-lag wall in David Wright's solar adobe (page 32). After sundown, heat begins to radiate from the wall to the house for twelve continuous hours, providing radiant heat. In the summer deciduous trees shade most of the wall, and much of the overhead sunlight is reflected off the glass. To aid in cooling, the upper vents in the Trombe wall are closed while the lower ones remain open. Four small fans at the top of the wall vented to the outside remove excess heat. This causes cooler air to be drawn into the open lower vents. If the windows on the north side of the house are open, then there is a net movement of cooler air across the house to these open vents. Venting the concrete wall to the outside at night cools it so that it can absorb heat from the rooms during the following day.

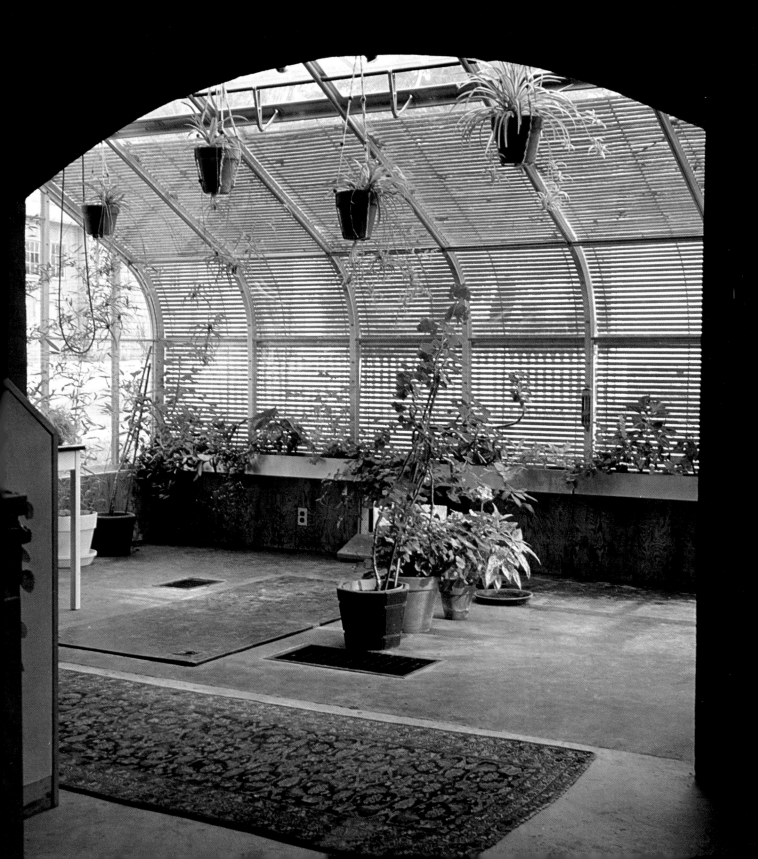

During the mild winter of 1975–76 Doug calculated that their house would consume about 39.6 cubic meters (1400 cubic feet) of natural gas for heating. Actual consumption was 9.6 cubic meters (338 cubic feet), or a savings of $108 based on local rates. Savings will certainly increase with more severe winters, but the point is that the house performed at 76 percent efficiency. (Had it been heated with electrical resistance heating, savings might have been as high as $800–900 per year.) That kind of energy savings was not the result of the Trombe wall alone. The remainder of the standard wood-frame house is heavily insulated (R20 in the walls and R40 in the ceiling) with cellulose fiber (recycled newspapers that have been fire- and insect-proofed). Around the outside perimeter to a depth of 60 centimeters (2 feet), 2.5 centimeters (1 inch) of Styrofoam insulation reduces subterranean heat loss. The windows on the north side provide for summer ventilation, thus further reducing unnecessary winter loss of heat.

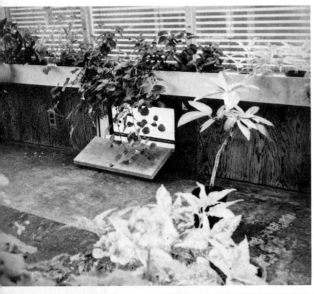

The greenhouse performs sympathetically with the Trombe wall, giving gains in direct heating to adjacent rooms and in latent heating as its thick concrete floor reradiates warmth to the living space above and the basement below. Vegetables and ornamentals in the greenhouse do not lend themselves to measurement by BTUs lost or gained. The greenhouse had to be double-glazed, to reduce heat loss, and shaded, to prevent overheating.

It is difficult to say where the solar system actually begins, but Doug has determined that about $8000 in additional costs are directly attributable to the solar devices. Based on accepted life-cycle analysis and a 5 percent annual inflation rate on natural gas, the solar components will be paid for in about seventeen years. An eleven-year amortization rate would be realized if the real cost of natural gas were to escalate at 15 percent per year. The real attraction of the system becomes apparent when one considers its life span: one hundred years. At the 5 percent inflation rate for fossil fuel, the Trombe will save $160,000 during its life.

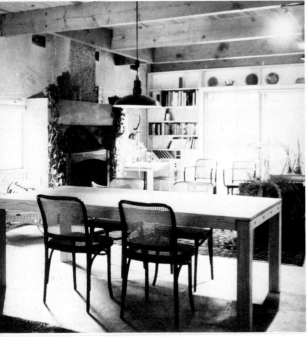

Perhaps the lifetime of the solar system might prove to be a more important economic factor than BTUs-per-dollar investment or collector efficiency. Free energy, like solar radiation, harnessed with inexpensive life-long passive systems, may mean that previous economic analyses were considering the wrong parameters. Whatever the future, the Kelbaughs now have a house that is simple to build, maintain, operate, and understand, which will conserve energy for a long time.

Saunders' Solar Shanty

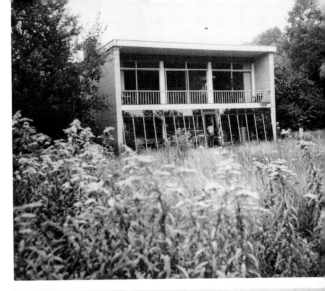

Weston, Massachusetts, is near America's birthplace so it is appropriate that one of the earliest pioneers of alternative energy should live there. Norman Saunders began to heat his home with solar energy in 1959, and since then, he has experimented with a number of different solar collectors, both passive and active. It is interesting to note that not one of the active flat-plate and concentrating collectors Mr. Saunders experimented with is still in use. He has come to favor almost totally passive heating and cooling systems.

The three acres of meadowland surrounding the Saunderses' home, appropriately named Experimental Manor, is an interesting climatological microcosm. The extremely cold winter temperatures mean that heating is much more important than cooling, and solar heating throughout the year has proved to be cost effective. Mr. Saunders has said that his house can maintain a temperature of 10° C. (50° F.) on a cloudy day in the dead of winter. Only a small amount of additional power from a backup system is necessary for additional heat.

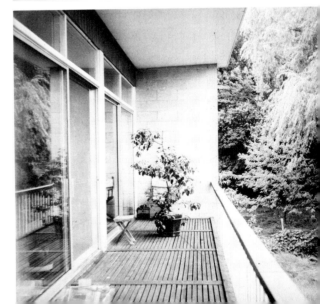

Experimental Manor is a 241-square-meter (2600-square-foot), two-story home. The north side of the first story is partially earth bermed, which keeps the house cooler in the summer and controls heat loss in the winter. The walls and floors are integral parts of the heating system. The first floor is a 15-centimeter (6-inch) concrete slab that absorbs heat from the sun during the day and re-radiates its warmth at night. The walls are massive—30-centimeter-(1-foot) thick—pumice blocks. Not only do these blocks serve as heat sinks, but because they have four times the thermal resistance of an ordinary block wall, they are also excellent insulators. Exploded mica has been added to the cavities in the blocks for further insulation. The ceiling is also heavily insulated, with the equivalent of 33 centimeters (13 inches) of fiberglass. That's a heat conservation of R57.5. To make better use of the house's thermal mass, a series of ducts with four separately operating fans circulates air. Three of the fans are used for general air circulation and warming, and a fourth recirculates room air to the floor ducts. This fan could be used in either heating or cooling modes.

The collector system is totally passive. Two-thirds of the entire south wall, 42.7 square meters (460 square feet), is glass. The lower floor is a single-glazed greenhouse that collects heat for the adjoining rooms. The second floor is a double-glazed series of sliding

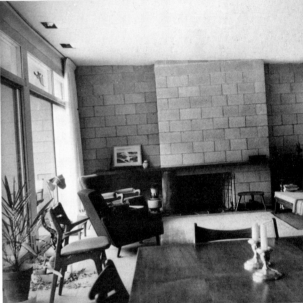

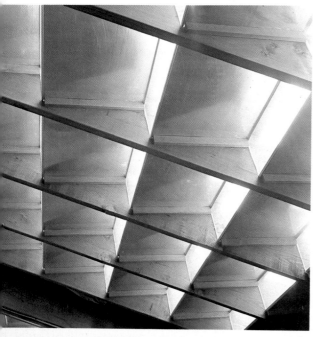

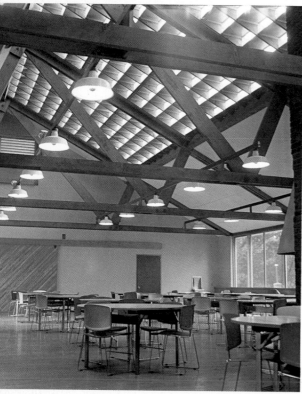

doors that open onto a darkly stained slatted deck. The massive walls and floors are heated by this glass, which receives direct sunlight. An unanticipated side benefit was gained from the second-floor deck: it is an effective heat collector, providing the entire heat load for the house in September and October.

How effective is such a straightforward solar system? The total heating needs are about 45,000 kilowatt-hours per year (1.54×10^8 BTUs per year). The south-facing windows collect 13,500 kilowatt-hours per year (4.6×10^7 BTUs per year), about 30 percent of the heating needs. At the very low rate of one cent per kilowatt-hour for natural gas, $135 can be saved each year by using this passive system. The system has long since paid for itself in the cost of fuel saved.

Twenty-seven years of research and sixteen years of active experimentation have given Norm Saunders the idea for a really interesting passive heating system. He has applied for a patent for his Solar Staircase (trademark) and has acted as consultant in its construction at the Cambridge School in Weston.

When the school's partially burned dining hall was being rebuilt, it was decided to include a solar system. Like Norm Saunders' home, the Cambridge School dining hall has great thermal mass. The north is of solid concrete block, is 30 centimeters (12 inches) thick, and is externally insulated with 10 centimeters (4 inches) of fiberglass. The south-facing wall is composed almost totally of glass, which furnishes both direct heat gain and a pleasing view. What really makes the building work, however, is the passive heat collector called the Solar Staircase.

The south-facing roof of the building is oriented about 27 degrees west of south. Compared to due south, this reduces heat collection by only a small percentage. Approximately 167 square meters (1800 square feet) of the 26-degree angled roof is a skylight covered with Filon, a corrugated fiberglass glazing. Under the Filon is a series of stairs treading their way up the roof. The tread of the stair is a lacquer-coated sheet of aluminum, 45 centimeters (18 inches) wide. The special lacquer minimizes corrosion and maintains maximum reflectivity, reducing the heat absorption of the aluminum. The risers are 21.5-centimeter (8½-inch) sheets of single-strength glass. This staircase arrangement provides a 15 percent energy saving on light alone. At night, upturned spotlights are directed toward the aluminum, giving excellent reflected light.

The staircase, which is in the school cafeteria, seems to have an effect on the students, who linger in this room longer than they did before the solar system was built. Perhaps its attraction lies in the combination of the unusual ceiling, diffuse natural light, and the ever-changing mottled patterns on the north wall. The vertical glass portion of the staircase allows the low-angled winter sun to enter the building for direct heat gain and to heat the massive north wall. The aluminum tread reflects additional radiation into the room, especially in winter. In the summertime when the sun is high overhead, the aluminum simultaneously shades and reflects.

The Cambridge School system is not complete. Norman Saunders' Solar Shanty, conveniently located between his home and the school, demonstrates the completed concept. It was constructed by a parent who was turned on to what Mr. Saunders was doing. The Shanty houses a series of 88-liter (22-gallon) translucent water-storage tanks called "heat radiators." These radiators are located under the staircase, parallel to the ground. In essence, they form a false ceiling. Directly beneath the radiators are rows of thermostated shutters. The sun pouring through the staircase heats the water in the radiators and provides direct heat to the spaces below. If the room is too warm, the shutters slowly close, isolating the radiators from the room. After sundown the room begins to cool and the shutters open, providing the room with gentle heat from what was stored in the water. Lights, similar to those in the school, give the same reflected illumination effects. (In hot weather this system can be used for cooling in a manner similar to that described for the house with the rooftop water beds, page 16.)

Without the heat radiators and shutters, the staircase costs $21.50 per square meter ($2 per square foot) more than a conventional roof. At present fuel prices—and based on the energy savings from this system—approximately $3 per square meter (28 cents per square foot) should be saved annually. This means a payoff period of seven years. Although more expensive, the complete Solar Staircase package will give great efficiency, and the return should not vary greatly from the figure cited. No monetary value can be placed on the additional stimulus of natural lighting and the pleasing architectural effects within a building incorporating the staircase.

Norman Saunders is confident of the practicality of his invention. It represents twenty-seven years of work, and he considers it the best of the many different collector systems he has tried.

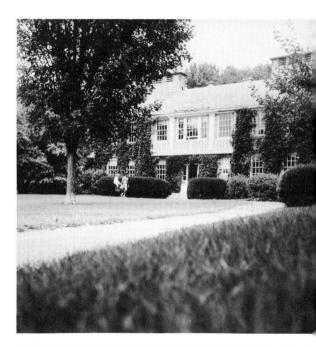

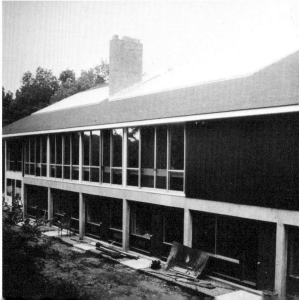

Total Environmental Action

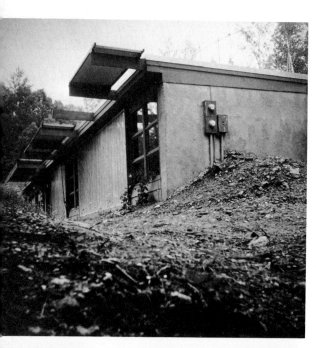

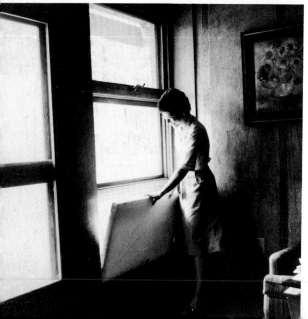

Total Environmental Action (TEA) is a group of young designers, researchers, and teachers with backgrounds in architecture who are involved in energy consultation, research and product development, and, especially, the creation of places in which to live and work that are in harmony with nature.

The area where the group operates, southern New Hampshire, is very cold. Though it is characterized by heavy snowfalls and below-freezing temperatures, the region does receive a considerable quantity of sunshine, and many people, like Ralph Tyrrell and Holly Anderson, have managed to capture this solar energy in TEA-designed houses. Ralph and Holly's house operates as a completely passive solar building, but it was not originally designed with that intention. In putting together this energy-conserving house, Doug Coonley and Bruce Anderson, two principal TEA designers, considered the thermal mass of the structure, its protection from the north wind, insulation and window positioning—and came up with an integrated design that had the least possible impact on the environment.

The north side of the house is buried to within a foot of the roof, so the cold north winds are directed over it. The entire house acts as a solar collector, like David Wright's Sunscoop (page 32). South-facing windows admit solar heat during the day, and heat is stored in the 10-centimeter (4-inch) concrete slab floor and concrete walls that are 20 centimeters (8 inches) to 30 centimeters (12 inches) thick. The heat is reradiated back to the house at night. The heat is prevented from escaping by 20 centimeters (8 inches) of fiberglass insulation in the ceiling and 5 centimeters (2 inches) of urethane foam on the north, east, and west exterior walls.

Unlike most solar collectors, which are mounted on the roof, these vertical panels are part of the building's south wall. Composed of two layers of Kalwall "Sunlite" Premium, a fiberglass-reinforced polyester sheet, they are positioned 7.5 centimeters (3 inches) apart, and cover a 2.7 × 10 meter (9 × 33 foot) section of the wall. Ten centimeters (4 inches) behind the interior layer of Kalwall is a painted black poured-concrete wall 30 centimeters (12 inches) thick. The arrangement and function of the two walls are very similar to those of the Trombe wall in the Kelbaugh residence (page 20), even to the vents in the top and bottom portions of the concrete wall. Originally the collectors were to be insulated with tiny poly-

26

styrene beads that would be blown between the Kalwall sheets when there was no sun and transferred to a storage drum in the garage by a 186-watt (¼-horsepower) blower during sunny periods, but it was found that the house functioned very well without the "Beadwall" addition.

Auxiliary heating is provided by the airtight heating stove or the wood-burning Styria cooking range. From September through March of 1975, only 2½ cords of wood were burned for cooking and heating.

Domestic hot water is preheated in a rather innovative manner. The cold-water supply line to the hot-water heater passes through about 23 meters (75 feet) of a 7.5-centimeter (3-inch) PVC pipe embedded in the concrete wall. The pipe has about 120 liters (30 gallons) of storage capacity. By turning down the thermostat to 44° C. (110° F.) and preheating the hot water with the sun, considerable savings in the electric hot-water heating system are realized.

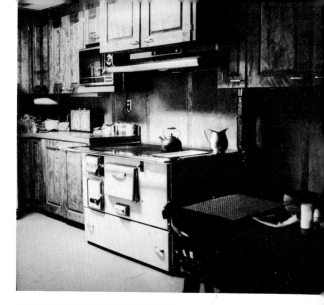

In this climate cooling is not a major problem, but when necessary, dampers on the north side of the house and in the concrete wall of the solar collector are opened to draw the cool air through the house and out of the collector. Removable overhangs cover the glass portion of the south wall. A number of deciduous trees facing the southern side of the building were preserved for natural shading. During the summer the house was kept between 20° C. (65° F.) and 24° C. (78° F.) by opening the windows whenever the outside temperature was lower than the inside. The action cools the thermal mass of the building, and the concrete absorbs excess heat from the house interior the following day. Ralph and Holly are very happy after their first year in the house; it has been using between 10 and 20 percent of the energy consumed for heating and cooling and heating water in the average New Hampshire home. The design alone reduces energy needs by about 45 percent over a conventional home. The added solar system meets about 75 percent of the remaining heat and hot-water energy needs. Here's a double-barreled approach to reducing energy costs—a properly designed house and a passive solar heating system.

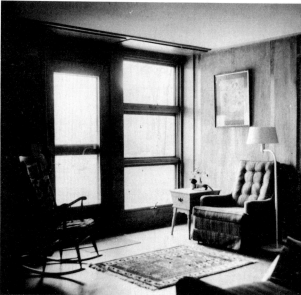

A final economic analysis tells the complete story of cost effectiveness. As of July 1975, final construction costs were $47,000, plus $5000 in design fees. This comes to $274 per square meter ($25.50 per square foot) for the 188-square-meter (2025-square-foot) house. Architect Doug Coonley estimates that the solar system added $6000 to the cost of the house, though real solar costs are hard to estimate in a house like this. The owners should easily recover the extra costs, and more, over the life of the mortgage.

A house that is designed on site for energy savings may reduce energy costs by as much as 50 percent. With this kind of incentive, one should have no difficulty in deciding what kind of house to build or what next summer's remodeling project will be. Evaluate your own personal situation, and if you can afford the few dollars more a solar system costs, why not go that route? But whatever you choose to do, either in retrofitting or in constructing a new home you can certainly afford to use the basic architectural techniques promoted by TEA.

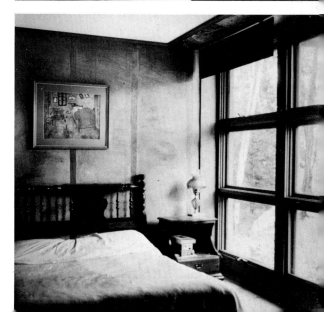

27

Carroll's Solar House for Normal People

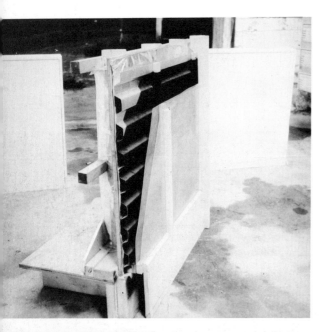

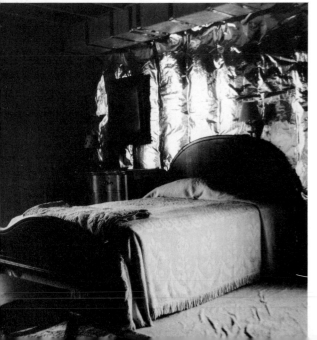

John Carroll is another on the growing list of environmental developers who are concerned with building cost-competitive houses that use little energy and appeal to home buyers. For instance, this 139-square-meter (1500-square-foot) rather conventional-looking house was built for a senior citizen in search of a home to which she could retire.

Carroll believes that the most cost-effective application that can be introduced into any home in cold central New Hampshire is insulation. A combination of fiberglass, ureaformaldehyde, and cellulose fiber was used to achieve a resistance factor of 22 in the walls and 45 in the ceiling. In fact, this house is so tightly constructed that heat loss is a low $5.9 \times 10\text{-}6$ kw/m2/hr (18.7 BTUs/ft2/hr.) when the temperature outside hits a very low of 18° C. (0° F.). Before construction begins, John builds models of parts of the house to determine how air will behave and how insulation will perform.

The house's heating mode has three independent systems: a solar system, an electrical system, and a wood stove. Solar energy is captured by a 48-square-meter (516-square-foot) vertical bank of Kalwall-glazed air collectors. The absorber plate is corrugated aluminum painted with Nextal, a selective coating. The corrugations of the plates run horizontally, and as air is heated it is drawn laterally across the plates to a maniford by a fan. This air is blown into a 36-kiloton (40-ton) river-rock storage bin under the house. Heating then takes place via a forced-air heater. Also embedded in the rock storage is a 120-liter (30-gallon) preheating heat exchanger for domestic hot water.

John likes this air system because the panels were simple to construct: three people worked two days to assemble them. These panels are lightweight. In New England, where there is much snow, weight on the roof must be minimal. One disadvantage of this arrangement is that the view to the south is completely blocked. John attempted to minimize this problem by breaking the collector bank and inserting a window in front of the dining-room table.

John Carroll is a thinking person's builder. For example, most builders in this area construct homes with an aluminum edge on the eaves, which is supposed to prevent ice dams from forming during extremely cold weather. The dams form, not because of large quantities of ice, but because of freeze-thaw cycles. The roof can be made to maintain consistent coolness with the construction of a continuous ridge vent to vent off excess heat. This prevents the

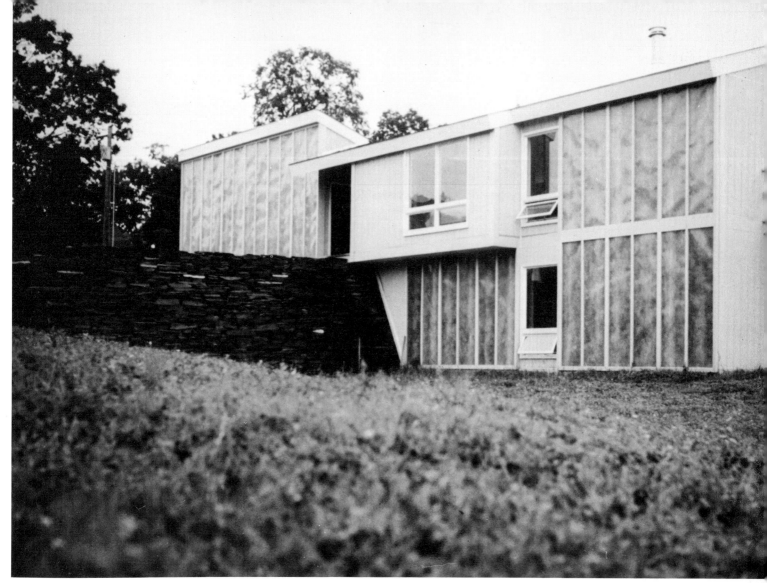

snow on the roof from melting and then refreezing and ice from accumulating.

A builder with a clear idea of needs of his region can perform long-range services for his clients and community. But no one person or single group of people can hope to convince the public that energy conservation is absolutely necessary. The federal government believes that a publicity campaign based on believable research is the only way people will be convinced that energy really is in short supply. If the government would look to the ideas of people like John Carroll, perhaps the necessity for energy conservation and the practical means by which it can be achieved could be demonstrated on a regional basis.

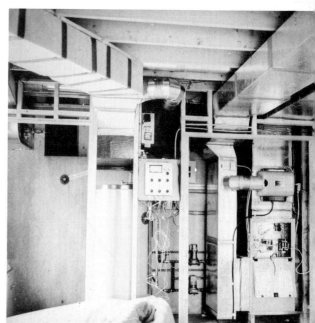

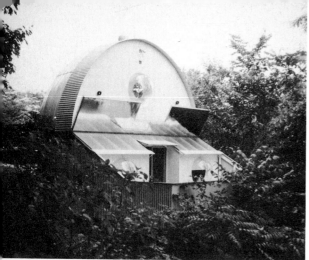

The Jantzens'
Collage of Sun Power

A number of alternative energy pioneers have not received proper recognition for their work simply because their rustic designs are alien to the general taste. The work of Mike Jantzen, an artist turned architect, and his wife Ellen, is both well engineered and esthetically acceptable. Their list of accomplishments is impressive. Among other projects, they have designed and constructed a solar water still, a solar sauna, three solar greenhouses, a solar-heated weekend cabin, and, during the summer of 1976, they began to build their own comprehensive alternative energy home.

Their largest completed project to date is a cabin built for Mike's parents. The two-story, 60-square-meter (650-square-foot) interior and 27-square-meter (290-square-foot) fenced sundeck are very functional ingredients of a vacation house. In addition, the price tag was practical: $10,000 covered all materials and appliances for the house and the cost of constructing the driveway. Labor costs were not a factor because they did all the work themselves.

Like so many solar-heated houses presently under construction, the Jantzen cabin is passively heated. The collectors, 11-square-meter (120-square-foot) panels glazed with corrugated Filon, are tilted at 30 degrees. This allows direct-heat gain through the transparent part of the roof. The glazed area is covered by an insulated reflector panel. A ship's winch and cable are used to hand-crank the panel open and closed. When opened to the proper angle, the reflector directs sun through the Filon into two 453-liter (120-gallon) water-storage tanks adjacent to the south wall. The tanks serve as thermal sinks; by turning over an insulated pad, they become bench seats. In the evening and during the summer the reflector panels are closed to reduce loss of heat. (A hinged desk top has been astutely placed beneath the staircase.)

The south wall looks as though it has three protruding bubbles. There is a 1.5-meter (5-foot) plastic bubble window on the second floor and two 1.2-meter (4-foot) bubbles flank the entrance on the ground floor. Windows of this type increase physical space, and more importantly, make the relatively small interior appear larger. They also focus light for direct-gain heating. At night and in the summer all three bubbles can be closed with insulated shutters.

The first-floor exterior is made up of painted steel siding. Fiberglass batt insulation is sandwiched in between a wood interior. The second floor is one-half the hemisphere of a silo top. When fitted together, the top and bottom floors, plus the sundeck, give the

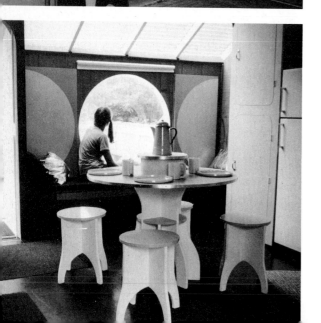

whole house a scoop effect. The southern orientation of the scoop enables the house to collect the winter sun. Because the house is painted white, it reflects much of the intense radiation from the high overhead summer sun. The half-silo has been sprayed with 5 centimeters (2 inches) of urethane foam insulation and then with Thermo-Gard fireproof paint.

All the furniture in the house was built by Mike. A green-topped kitchen table is novel in that the center cylinder supports a built-in light, which eliminates the need for an overhead fixture and also aids in keeping foods warm. Vertical wall-mounted fluorescent lights in the kitchen blend in well with the interior design and also conserve energy.

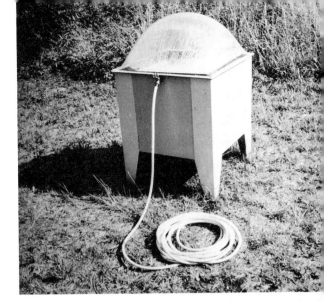

At this point, Mike and Ellen don't know how much energy the house will conserve. One experiment proved that they were able to get the inside temperature to 37° C. (98° F.) on a sunny day when the temperature outside was only —15° C. (5° F.). Venting and shading will prevent overheating. The major problem, Mike notes, is that the heat-storage system provides only one evening's carryover in a cold winter, but then, this is a vacation house used mainly in the summer.

The solar still that Mike designed and built has produced up to 3.5 liters of potable water in a day. The hose is attached to the domestic water supply. Water is run into a shallow pan heated by the sun. The evaporated water then condenses on the plastic dome cover and the distilled water runs down the sides of the dome and still into a storage container. A faucet at the rear of the still provides instant pure water. The still is attractive enough so that most people would not object to having it occupy a spot on their sun porch.

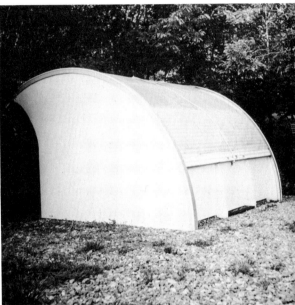

Ellen has three gardens that occupy much of her time. A greenhouse extends the growing season and gives more latitude on plant varieties that can be grown. In the winter of 1974–75 the electrical heating costs for a noninsulated greenhouse were between $50 and $60 per month. Mike decided that he could reduce heating costs with insulation. From October 1975 to March 1976 the cost for electricity in an insulated greenhouse with a solar storage system was $24.70. In addition to being energy efficient, the greenhouses are architecturally appealing. The larger greenhouse has a rock storage system on the north wall. Two important features of this greenhouse are the sliding, corrugated, insulated fiberglass covers and the excellent use of north-wall space. Since the north wall of any greenhouse is only a source of heat loss in the winter, it makes more sense to completely insulate this area. Mike did this, but continued the arch of the Quonset-shaped building into an overhang. The overhang serves as a work-storage space.

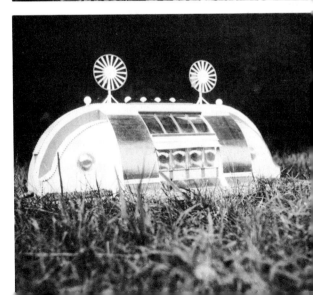

The Jantzens' current endeavor is their own house, and what a house it will be—as the model illustrates. Integrate the ideas of a person who is knowledgeable about energy (Mike) with those of a person who has studied biology and food production (Ellen), and the result should be interesting, to say the least. The finished house will incorporate energy-conserving principles, conceptual spaces, and green belts, and exemplify the Jantzens' respect for their environment.

The Wright Way

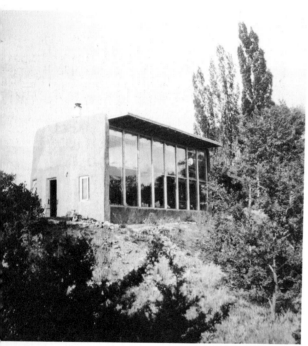

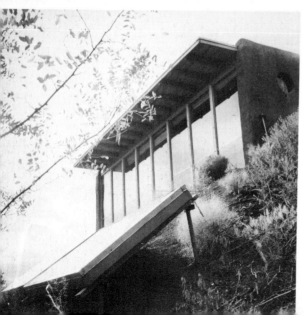

Few people associated with home building are producing houses that complement the landscape. Perhaps loan institutions, contractors, or would-be residents are dictating the style of homes that are being built. There is, however, a small number of progressive architects dedicated to designing homes that are in tune with both their surroundings and the life-styles of the people who live in them. David Wright, an environmental architect whose initial contributions were in solar adobe construction in New Mexico, is one such architect. The two Wright-designed houses in Santa Fe, New Mexico, are evidence of a pleasing regional architecture that can be maintained using passive solar applications.

The climatic conditions of northern New Mexico should be explained. This area is a semidesert that receives only about 30 centimeters (12 inches) of rain per year, and it is also quite cold. For example, Santa Fe is at an elevation of just under 650 meters (7000 feet) and has an annual snowfall of 80 centimeters (31.5 inches). The city usually has more than ten days of below-zero temperatures during the winter. Heating and extending the growing season are prime concerns of the people living in this area.

David's first energy-conserving house was completed in the fall of 1974. Clark and Charlotte Kimball are now living in the very open one-and-one-half story house they call Sunscoop. The long axis of this adobe house runs east to west. A series of vertical two-story windows that constitutes an area of 37 square meters (400 square feet) is located on the house's south side. These windows scoop the low, 30-degree-angled winter sun and provide direct-gain solar heating to the entire house, except for the entrance foyer. Though the windows act simply as passive solar collectors, many other features have been designed into the house to make them work.

The walls of the house are massive, varying from 33 to 43 centimeters (13 to 17 inches) thick. They serve as heat-lag heat sinks; heated by the sun during the day, they reradiate that heat into the living space throughout the night. Adobe has a time lag of about 12 hours per 30 centimeters (12 inches) of thickness, which means that heat is continually radiated during that time period. The heat is prevented from escaping to the outside by 5 centimeters (2 inches) of exterior Styrofoam insulation. The insulation is covered with adobe cement, and earth is bermed from the floor level to about a height of 1 meter (39 inches) on the north wall. In a recent interview with *Adobe News* David compared the house to a thermos bottle. Like a thermos, the house is externally insulated to check heat loss. Even the south-facing windows have hinged insulated shutters that can be lowered to prevent loss of heat. A banco that can serve as a chair, bed, or just a place to lounge runs the length of the south wall just inside and below the windows. Adobed into this banco are 220-liter (55-gallon) water-filled drums for additional heat-storage capacity. In the evening this area is ideal for sitting and watching the night sky. Sunscoop's water and adobe mass has a tempering effect on the temperature behavior of the house during winter. In March 1975 the minimum and maximum outside temperatures ranged from —15° C. to 13° C., respectively (5° F. to 56° F.); the downstairs house temperature fluctuated between an average low of 13.4° C. (56° F.) and a high of 20.2° C. (68° F.). The lowest temperature was 10° C. (50° F.). These temperatures were maintained without benefit of backup heating, and although they sound a bit low, the house feels comfortable because heat is radiated from the walls, floors, and bancos.

David also installed a thermosiphon solar hot-water heating system. On the south side of a hill below the house he set up two 10-square-meter (105-square-foot) collector panels inclined at 45 degrees. The collector is plumbed to a large insulated tank in the closet of the house. The sun-heated water flows to the tank in the house by convective currents, and, in the same way, flows back to the collector when it is cool. A standard hot-water heater inside the tank picks up heat for domestic purposes. Nine months out of twelve hot water is free, compliments of the sun, and about 50 percent of the hot water used during the winter is sun-heated.

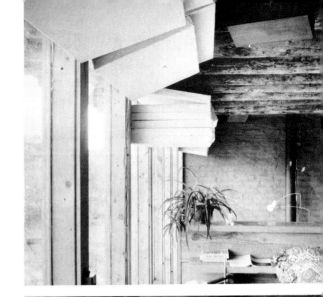

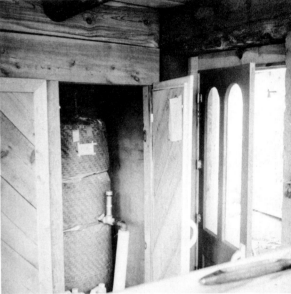

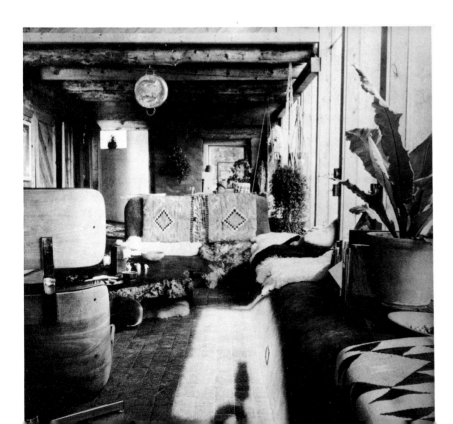

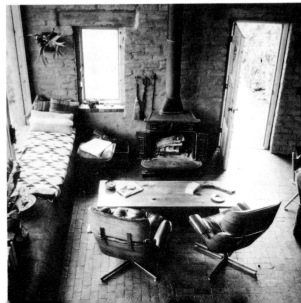

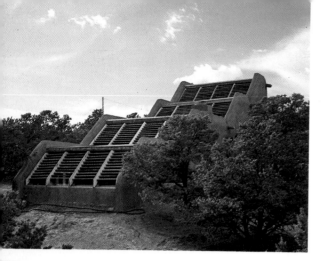

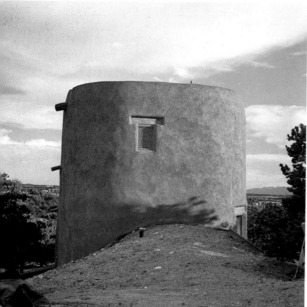

Whereas the mass provides tempering during the winter, shading—a 1.2-meter (4-foot) overhang on the south side—provides cooling during the summer. Wright's only criticism is that these shades should have been made more maneuverable to shield the house from sun during the fall when sunlight is at a lower angle.

Karen Terry is living in a David Wright passive sun-tempered solar-designed home that she, with a small boost from friends, built *herself*. The credit for design should actually go to a group of eleventh-century Indians who built Pueblo Bonito in Chaco Canyon, New Mexico, and Montezuma's Castle in northeastern Arizona. These early Americans practiced solar orientation just to keep warm; they hardly had to worry about saving energy. Karen's 89-square-meter (960-square-foot) house stair-steps down the south-facing slope of a hill in an almost ideal site-oriented fashion. The four banks of double-paned windows are the basis for the passive solar system. These 45-degree sloped windows cover 37 square meters (400 square feet) of the southern roof and allow the winter sun in to warm the heat-sink areas, which are similar to those in the Sunscoop. Karen, with the help of Jerry Yudelson from California's Office of Appropriate Technology, designed a series of two-by-six slats to fit across the skylight windows for shading in the summertime. The slats are removed manually at the onset of winter. Karen will eventually construct insulated shutters to cover the collector-glass area, but she's in no hurry to do this because even with the heat loss through these windows, she needed no extra heat during the winter of 1975. The living spaces are arranged according to the principle that heat stratifies and rises. The lowest level, which is the coolest, is the area of greatest activity, and serves as a workshop. The middle area supports the kitchen and living room. At the top, which is the warmest part of the house, are the bathroom and loft bedroom.

The auxiliary heating system consists of an adobe fireplace and a small wood-burning stove. The thermos-bottle principle is strictly adhered to. The adobe walls are covered on the outside by 5 centimeters (2 inches) of rigid polyurethane, followed by black felt, wire mesh, and stucco. The ceiling is likewise insulated with polyurethane. Earth is bermed up on the east, west, and north walls. The floors were dug 60 centimeters (2 feet) into the earth, and a plastic moisture barrier was laid. Then 5 centimeters (2 inches) of styrene insulation was placed on the barrier, and the 60 centimeters of earth was replaced. Adobe bricks are the actual floor.

On the day we visited Karen, the great New Mexico sky was performing at its best. The cerulean blue background and billowy white clouds provided a sculptured backdrop for the gentle lines of the house, which I'll call the "canted sunstrip." Inside and out, throughout the day the house responded to the changing sun angles and intensity with exquisite patterns and colors. With pride, Karen can reflect that she has composed a home that is in tune with the environment. It serves as an example for others to follow and has given her the necessary experience to build other energy-effective homes, one of which is now under construction.

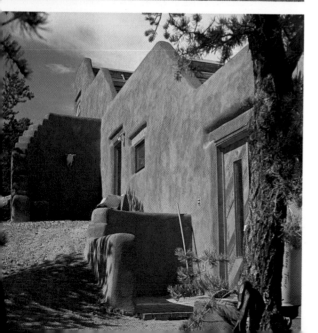

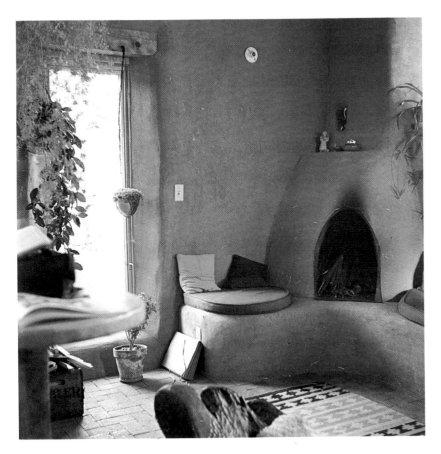

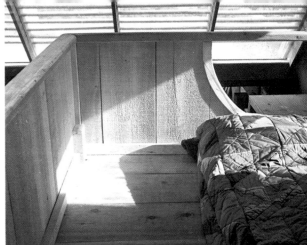

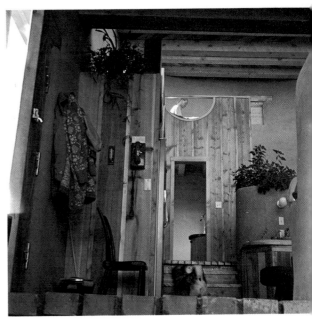

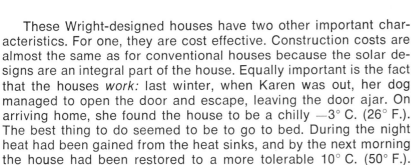

These Wright-designed houses have two other important characteristics. For one, they are cost effective. Construction costs are almost the same as for conventional houses because the solar designs are an integral part of the house. Equally important is the fact that the houses *work:* last winter, when Karen was out, her dog managed to open the door and escape, leaving the door ajar. On arriving home, she found the house to be a chilly —3° C. (26° F.). The best thing to do seemed to be to go to bed. During the night heat had been gained from the heat sinks, and by the next morning the house had been restored to a more tolerable 10° C. (50° F.).

David Wright theorizes that, to be successful, a passive solar adobe house should be oriented to the sun, flexible enough to accommodate all seasons, insulated, appropriately engineered as to mass, glazing location, and size, livable and functional—and visually pleasing. He notes that housing construction is similar throughout the United States, even though there are vast climatological and geographical differences.

David Wright represents the new breed of architect who can help lead us to sensitive kinds of construction that deal effectively with regional differences and natural environments.

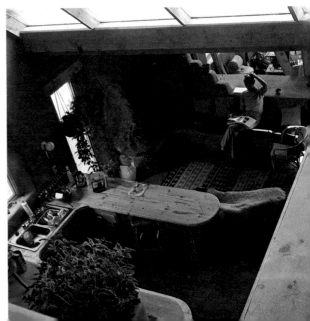

The Solarizing of Coos Bay

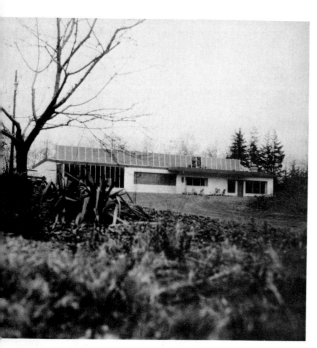

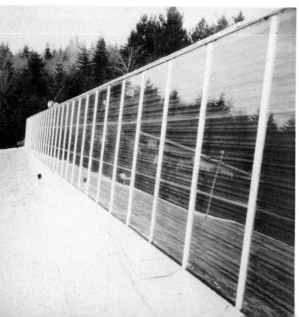

John Reynolds, an instructor of architecture at the University of Oregon, was surprised to learn that someone had built a solar house in Coos Bay, Oregon. Coos Bay's frequent fogs made it seem an unlikely place for the use of solar energy.

In 1967 Henry Mathew designed and built this home that is located 8.5 kilometers (5 miles) from the ocean in an area characterized by between 112.5–225 centimeters (45–90 inches) of annual rainfall. There is intermittent fog and mist between October to May, but fog may roll in at any time of the year. Henry was undaunted, and after experimenting with a smaller home, he built this one.

Architecturally the house is very straightforward. It is a single-story, 151-square-meter (1624-square-foot) structure whose long axis is oriented east to west, with an attached garage and greenhouse of the same size. The most striking features are the 37 square meters (400 square feet) of almost vertical panels located on top of the house. There are an additional 32.5 square meters (350 square feet) of free-standing panels to the north of the house. Mr. Mathew built the panels himself from corrugated black-painted aluminum sheets laced with 13-millimeter (½-inch) galvanized iron pipe and covered with a single layer of glass. Water is pumped through these pipes by a ¼-horsepower pump at about 17 gallons per minute to the heart of the heating system—a huge 32,000-liter (8000-gallon) insulated thin-gauge steel storage tank located under the house. Thermostatically controlled dampers regulate the flow of hot air from the storage tank through a large homemade baffled vent near the ceiling on the east side of the living room. The indirectly solar-heated air moves into the living areas by gravity convection currents. A second vent across the living room in the fireplace hearth revolves the cooled air back to the solar hot-water tank.

The roof of the house is truly unusual. It cost only $80 and complements the solar collection. Plastic roofing cement was painted on the roof, and heavy-duty aluminum foil was unrolled into the cement while it was still tacky. The additional light directed to the collectors by this roof increases collector efficiency about 30 percent. Furthermore, the roof has surprising longevity. When I visited Mr. Mathew, the north side of his foil-covered roof was nine years old and still in good shape, even though roofs that support solar panels tend to get more foot traffic than the average roof. One additional note is that the 8-degree sloping and the vertical collectors work well together. Mr. Mathew feels that with the sun at a 32-degree angle in winter, vertical collectors are most efficient.

The materials for the entire system cost $1300 in 1967. The system has paid for itself about three times over through reduced energy costs. The active plus the passive aspects of the Mathew solar house satisfy about 90 percent of the heating needs. The windows on the south side of the house are responsible for meeting about 22 percent of the winter heating needs through direct-gain heating. This reinforces the premise that orientation to site and proper design will take care of most needs; the active system is often like the extras we buy for cars. It must be admitted, though, that in the Pacific Northwest active systems provide a greater percentage of energy needs than in sunnier climates. The behavior of the large storage tank demonstrates the usefulness of an active system on the Oregon coast.

In 1975 the storage tank was up to 68° C. (155° F.), a maximum. On a bright sunny day the tank temperature will increase by 5.5° C. (10° F.). That's about 1,000,000 BTUs of energy. On cold days when ambient air temperatures are about —4° C. (25° F.), the tank will decay about 2° C. (4° F.) in a day. The point is that this large tank provides sufficient storage capacity to allow for the less dependable coastal sunshine.

With relatively little help from others, and an adverse climate to contend with, Henry Mathew did what we are trying to convince people to do for themselves in *Living with Energy.* He is ahead of most of us, but efforts such as his are illustrating how to live within the perimeters of our available energy.

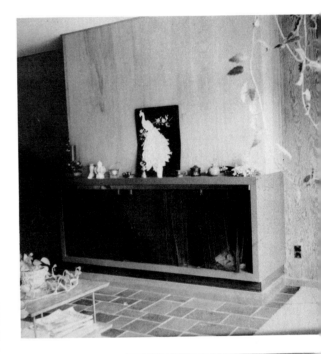

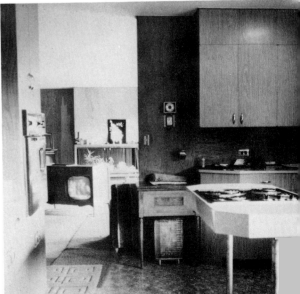

37

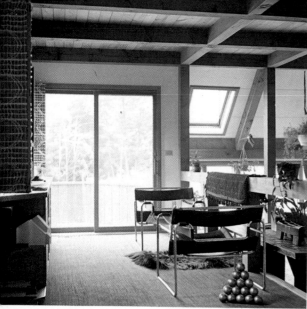

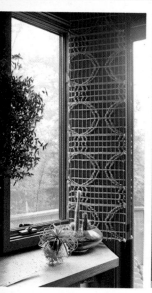

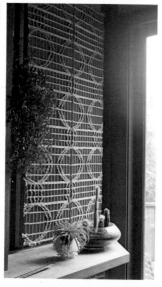

Sunstream Energy House

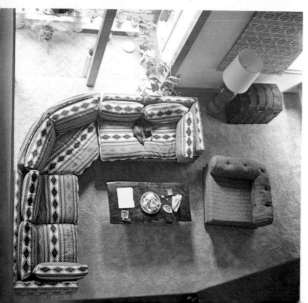

The south roof of Energy House at Quechee Lake, Vermont, is 37 square meters (400 square feet) of roll-bond absorber plates in two 45-degree-angled banks. The convex, self-cleaning, no-glare acrylic-glazed panels provide a delightful modishness that the more common flat-plate collectors do not. The house was designed by Blue Minges of Blue-Sun Ltd. and was built by its owner, Robert Terrosi.

The architect's prime considerations in designing this 223-square-meter (2400-square-foot), two-and-one-half-story house were the harshness of the Vermont climate and the high cost of fuel in this area. Compare the energy costs of this house with those of a more conventional home. The solar system cost an additional $7000 over normal construction, but lower annual expenditures for energy mean that, compared to an an all-electric system, the solar hardware will pay for itself in four and a half years, and compared to an oil-heated house with electrically heated water, it will pay for itself in eleven and a half years. A scaled-down heating system would, of course, be less expensive, but payoff periods would be about the same.

Two aspects of the Energy House are intriguing. One is the use of the heat pump in combination with a solar system. The other is the low temperatures at which everything functions. The heat pump works in the following manner: Heat from the outside, in this case air that has been warmed by being blown across coils of solar-heated water, is used to evaporate Freon, which picks up heat from the air. An electrical compressor raises the pressure on the now-vaporized Freon and allows it to condense in tubes exposed to inside air. As the Freon condenses, it releases heat. This heat energy in turn raises the temperature of the fan-pumped air flowing through a forced-air heating system. Heat pumps work more efficiently in temperatures of about 10° C. (50° F.) to 15° C. (60° F.), but their average efficiency is measured by a coefficient of performance (COP) rating. For example, a COP means that there are three units of heat-energy output for each unit of electrical-energy input.

Since the heat pump works best at lower temperatures, the solar panels only collect water up to 27° C. (80° F.). This low-

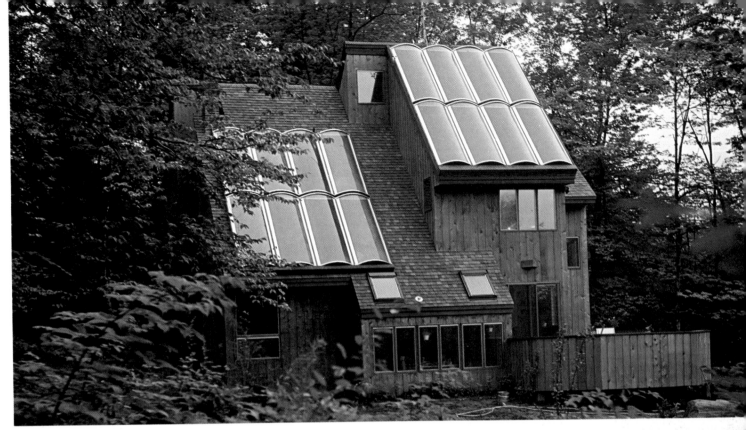

temperature operation enables the collectors to operate more efficiently because there is less heat loss to the atmosphere— that is, the temperature difference between the air and the solar system is not large. When the mixture, a 50–50 combination of ethylene glycol and water, in the 9600-liter (2400-gallon) insulated storage tank reaches 27° C., then the solar domestic hot-water system is activated. About 54 percent of hot-water needs are provided in this manner.

Bob Terrosi regards these solarwares as the gravy for the real meat and potatoes of energy conservation: the design of the house. Like any low-energy-use structure, the house is heavily insulated and tightly sealed with weatherstripping. All windows are triple glazed for an even greater reduction in heat loss. The skylight windows at the "top of the stack" were imported from Denmark and can be opened and closed from the first floor for ventilation. Most windows are kinetically insulated with colorful urethane shutters.

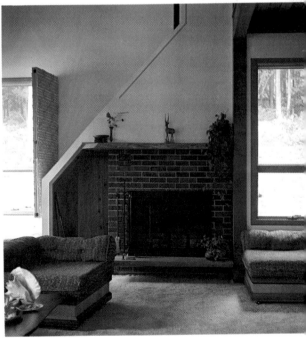

In addition, prevailing southwest summer winds entering through windows on that side of the house are vented out through the skylight windows on the northeast roof. This chimney effect enables the house to be cooled with natural air currents. A vestibule entrance acts as an airlock to reduce heat loss, and the solarium on the south wall is not only decorative but also furnishes additional heat through direct solar gains.

From the windbreak of tall trees on the north to the sun-accepting transparency on the south, the Energy House is a combination of passive and active strategies that reap the sunny benefits of energy conservation.

Alten Associates Assignment: Project Survival

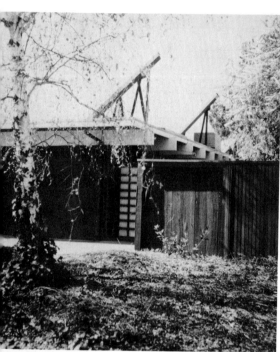

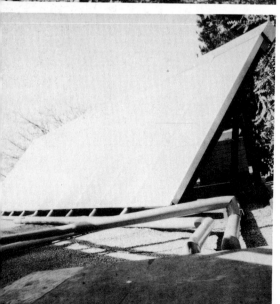

Alten Associates of Mountain View, California, designs and retrofits homes to be energy efficient. The organization, which gained its impetus from a parent group called Project Survival, began as a nonprofit advisory body of people with technical backgrounds who had a common interest in less polluting forms of energy. When two members—one of them president Klaus Heinemann—retrofitted their homes, community interest in Alten projects began to increase, and it was decided to establish an office and develop a full-time staff, yet maintain a nonprofit status. Today Alten is helping to set the stage for more widespread adoption of alternative energy.

Before Alten retrofitted the Winston Boone residence in Palo Alto, California, the home was thoroughly insulated with Monotherm. Monotherm is a product of conservation efforts: recycled newspaper is insect- and fire-proofed and puffed into a fluffy material that can either be blown into the attic or placed in the walls. A do-it-yourself material, Monotherm has better insulation values than fiberglass.

The roof was flat, and in order to gain greater efficiency in the solar collectors at this latitude, it was necessary to tilt the panels to a 45-degree angle. The angled panels are made less conspicuous by the surrounding trees. As there is greater solar intensity during the afternoons in this part of California, it was desirable to orient collector panels slightly west of south.

Marketed under the name of Olin Roll Bond, the panels are made of copper tube and aluminum fin and are covered with Tedlar. This glazing increases the efficiency of the panels' manifold by preventing the captured long-wave radiation from being re-radiated—the much-storied "greenhouse effect."

The water that is pumped through the collectors is stored in a cylindrical 8000-liter (2000-gallon) underground tank, which has been insulated so it will not lose its stored heat to the earth. The earth is not a good insulator but does temper the climate. Polyurethane was the insulation used in this case, but a less expensive material could have been used if the tank had been placed indoors. From the tank, the heated water is pumped to the house where a can-coil system functions as a forced-air heater. The result is that about 80 percent of all heating needs are met by this sun-energized heater. The existing gas heater was tied in for backup.

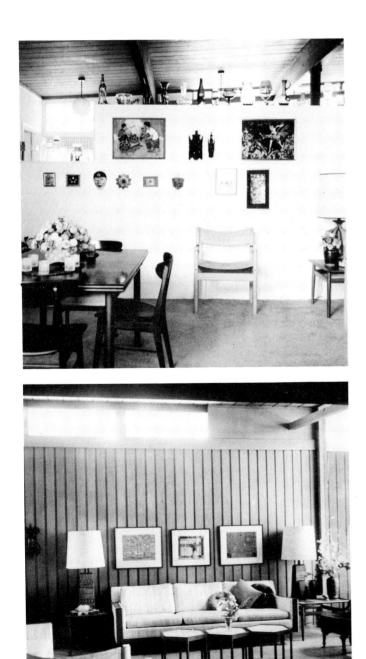
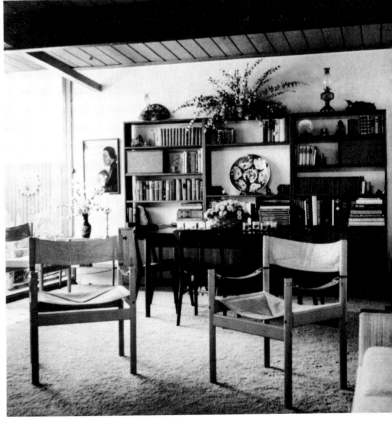

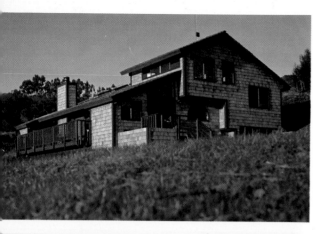

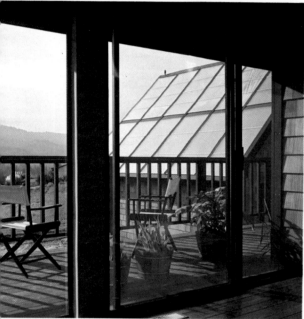

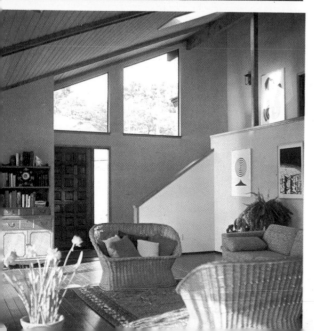

Surprisingly enough, it is impossible to tell the difference between heat that is provided by the sun and that from natural gas. The one thing that becomes evident is that living in a sun-heated house really *feels* better.

Alten's long-range goal is to develop a low-cost kit for solarizing existing homes. Since harvesting the sun's energy is not a highly technical process, Alten believes in the practicality of the do-it-yourself approach.

Phil and Bobbie Barry of Portola Valley were the benefactors of a solar home designed by Alten Associates. The Barrys built their house as a political statement against nuclear power plant construction. In fighting California's Nuclear Plant Initiative in 1976, Phil and Bobbie opened their house to the public to show that solar power works—it's beautiful and it's functional. They feel that promoting conservation through government tax incentives would be a safer, saner way to help meet energy needs. Their 232-square-meter (2500-square-foot) luxurious dwelling nestled in the California Coast Range is unique because the sun-harvesting system has been placed on the adjacent garage rather than the roof of the house. This allows for more flexibility in house design and orientation and also "conceals the fact that the house is solar heated." Of course, some basic principles of solar design do limit building freedom. One disadvantage of the Barrys' arrangement is that it is more expensive to operate because it requires additional plumbing materials and a larger pump.

Otherwise, the solar system is relatively conventional. There is an 8000-liter (2000-gallon) insulated hot-water storage tank in the basement. The 36 square meters (384 square feet) of Tedlar-covered Olin Roll Bond collector panels are plumbed to the tank, which in turn is plumbed to a heat exchanger. The house is heated when air is blown across the hot pipes of the exchanger and feeds a conventional forced-air system. Air conditioning is not necessary. A heat pump serves as a backup system, and this device saves about 50 percent in energy costs compared to the typical electrical system in this area.

The Barry house is beautiful: a large living area looks out over the mountains and the home's four half-levels provide all five Barrys with private space. Here is an esthetically designed home with a solar system that will pay for itself in eight to ten years.

Solar designs are practical in funky mountain cabins and opulent mansions, and everything in between. One HUD study admitted that 40 percent of all housing in the United States will be solar-powered by 1990. But the time for positive action is now.

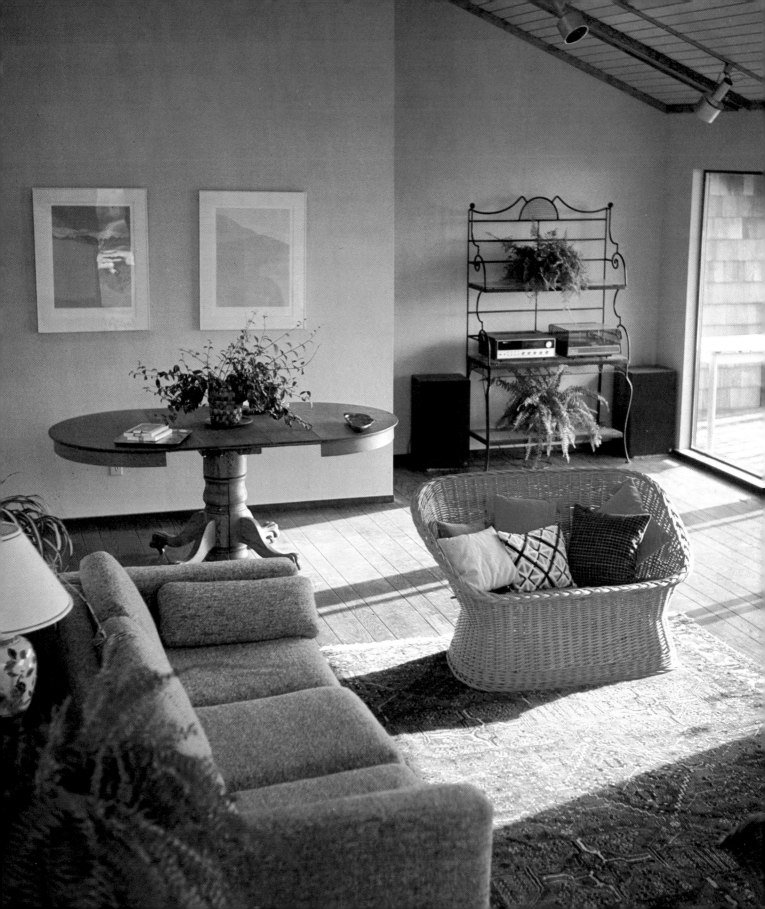

The Metaphysical Gymnasium

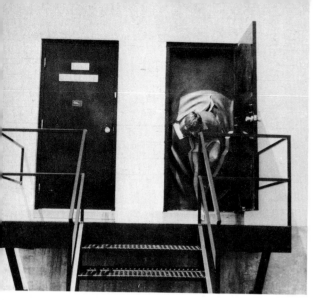

Mr. Future, attired in his simcoll-covered sun-absorbing jumpsuit, slides through the sphincter door to his modularized metaphysical gymnasium. The activities of a space person on some far-off planet? Not quite. However, Ted Bakewell III's terra firma ideas may well be the prototypes for our future life-styles. Ted lives in a warehouse in St. Louis, Missouri, and uses old scaffolds, cardboard barrels, and piles of sponge rubber as part of his furniture. Sounds bizarre, but by using recycled, low-cost materials, Bakewell is developing practical ideas for homes and life-styles of the future.

Ted has chosen to live in the warehouse he calls his metaphysical gymnasium because it enables him to work out ideas that are directed toward helping people meet their housing needs. His total design concept is an attempt to better utilize materials that are now being wasted. "Conservation" is his byword, and Ted's home is a demonstration model. Because it is a warehouse and uses old business wares, "industrial camping" is an appropriate description of its operation.

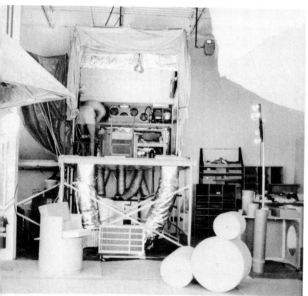

From the outside the warehouse doesn't look quite normal: the protruding Plexiglas window and dissected sponge-rubber door are quite remarkable. The Plexiglas bubble faces the southeast and concentrates the low winter sun for direct-gain morning warmth. The sponge-rubber door, dubbed the "sphincter door," would be ideal for families with kids because going through it is such fun. Its automatic quick-closing action conserves heat.

If the outside of Ted's place arouses curiosity, the inside is even more fascinating. The large room has been modularized into a series of living spaces. The "sluterus" (slinky uterus), a nylon sheet with a series of equally spaced plastic pipes in casings can be pushed against the wall and hooked for convenient out-of-the-way storage, or accordioned out and transformed into a comfortable lounge or evening entertainment room. Note the net bag, filled with scrap pieces of Styrofoam, which serves as a lounge. The three cloth-covered tubes in the foreground are held together with recycled seat belts—an incredibly comfortable chair.

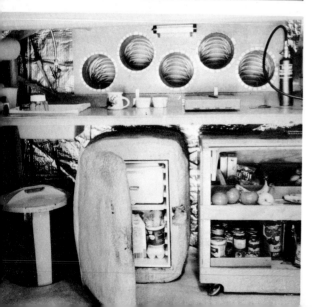

On the way to the kitchen/bathroom module you pass a recycled butcher's cart that serves as an excellent portable stereo cabinet. There's also a cardboard barrel that has been fashioned into a chair and an umbrella lampshade that creates pleasant diffused light from the upturned spotlight.

At first glance the kitchen/bathroom consists of yellow and blue awnings sitting atop a scaffold. These awnings can close off the area, which is heated by a small portable heater. The two silver tubes under the yellow awning are ducts from the heater to the kitchen. Energy conservation in this arrangement is self-evident. The kitchen has all kinds of little Bakewellisms. A small icebox is completely insulated with urethane foam on the outside. Ted renews the ice about once each week. Next to the icebox is a portable cupboard that can be rolled out, the leaves turned down, and presto!—four people can dine comfortably. In the wall behind the sink and drainboard are five openings. Here is a most incredible energy-conserving disposal. Tubes lead down to five recycling bins for organic materials, glass, steel, paper, and aluminum.

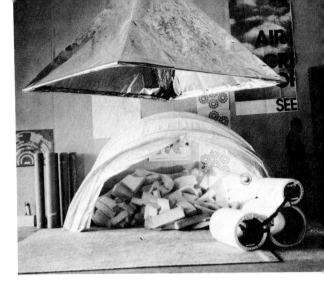

The bathroom likewise conserves energy. Here a ship's toilet saves both water and energy, though Ted thinks that a small composting toilet is a more practical waste-recycle alternative. His shower uses a water-conserving pressure head. The water is pressurized by a hand pump, enabling the user to get some exercise before each shower, and only five liters of water are used per shower. The water from the shower and sinks is never really used up because it's collected in a small cistern and pumped to the roof where a solar still makes it reusable. Water for showering and washing is heated by a very small electrical heating device on the end of the shower tube. These heaters are manufactured in Italy and Brazil and are in wide use in many Third World countries.

A recycled triple-tiered scaffold has been retrofitted to accommodate Ted's clothes on the bottom tier; office space, complete with desk, chair, and filing cabinet, in the middle; and a bed at the top, the warmest level. If he wants to do paperwork before retiring, Ted simply lowers a nylon tube over the whole arrangement and hooks up the heater at the base.

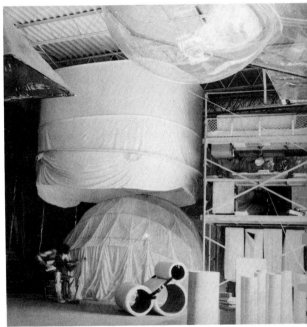

The metaphysical gym is only a weekend and evening activity. During the day Ted works for Bakewell Corporation, a building and development firm owned by his father. He admits that his influence in the building of shopping centers is not as great as he would like it to be. However, one of his ideas has been used in a shopping area in the Ladue section of St. Louis, Missouri: parking spaces of alternating concrete squares and soil. The grass allowed to grow in the parking lot cools the asphalt jungle. Water runoff following rains is also reduced, because some moisture penetrates the soil. Ted's ultimate plan is to actualize his inventions and ideas in a house for himself. In the meantime, he will continue to experiment at his home in the warehouse.

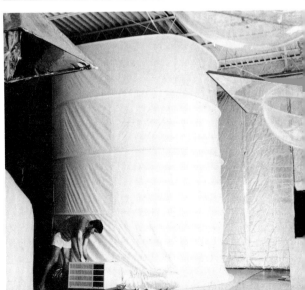

45

Quigley's Kinetic Architecture

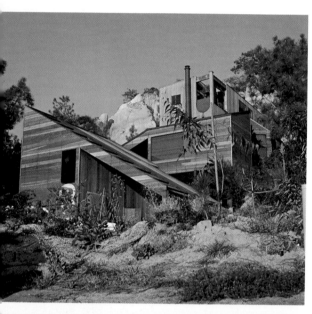

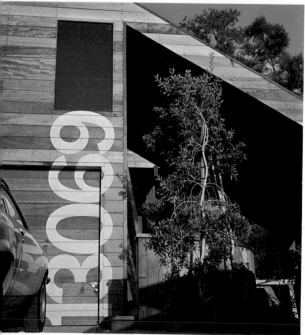

Western San Diego County is blessed with one of the most mellow climates in the United States. Temperature fluctuations are slight, and the sun shines almost throughout the year. Life there can be made even more comfortable if the climatic fluctuations are smoothed out. A benign climate makes it somewhat easier to use natural energy sources for house heating and cooling, and water heating. However, the use of alternative energy in home construction is only half the battle, according to architect Rob Quigley of San Diego.

Rob's approach to architecture is total. A house is more than just a place in which to live. Quigley feels that a house should be conceived and constructed to fit the living and working styles of its occupants. In order to understand the real needs and desires of a potential client, he holds a series of sessions with the future home owner. In his "psychohomalysis," Rob attempts to discover how a client lives, what he and his family want to do in their home, and what they want their home to do for them. This information, coupled with an understanding of the site limitations where the home is to be built, enables Rob to develop a design. He feels that designing a house should not be an architectural ego trip, even though it may seem impossible for an architect to remove himself from his design completely.

Irrespective of its energy-conservation applications, Andy and Flossy Cohen's house is a work of "art-titecture." The house won the honor award in San Diego County's 1976 American Institute of Architecture competition. Inside and out the Cohen home is a magnificent, ever-changing visual experience. Andy and Flossy have gathered art treasures from Japan, Bali, Ethiopia, Central America, and the Philippines, and other places. Flossy periodically changes these works of art, many of which are worthy of exhibition in a museum, and adds her own work. The natural kinetic changes in the art forms created by the sun's travel make the experience complete. Rob pointed out that the natural lighting changes designed into the house were not accidental. He noted that NASA has documented the fact that changes in a person's living space are necessary to maintain mental health. The Cohen house is a healthy environment.

Charles Milligan has captured one feature of this home that deserves emphasis—site design. The lot was a triangular 1350 square meters (⅓ acre) and was bounded on two sides by tortuous sand-

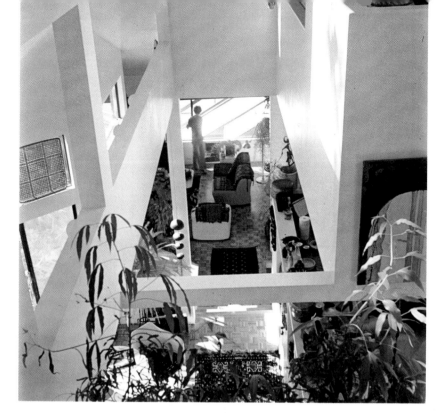

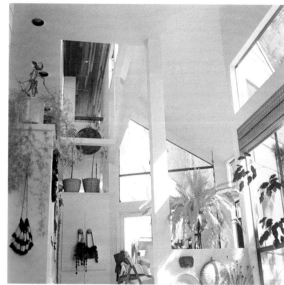

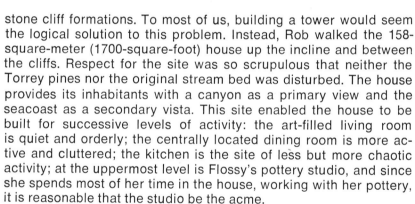

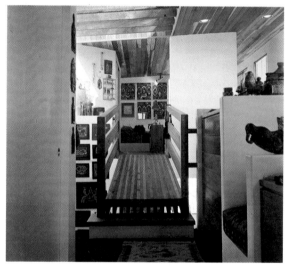

stone cliff formations. To most of us, building a tower would seem the logical solution to this problem. Instead, Rob walked the 158-square-meter (1700-square-foot) house up the incline and between the cliffs. Respect for the site was so scrupulous that neither the Torrey pines nor the original stream bed was disturbed. The house provides its inhabitants with a canyon as a primary view and the seacoast as a secondary vista. This site enabled the house to be built for successive levels of activity: the art-filled living room is quiet and orderly; the centrally located dining room is more active and cluttered; the kitchen is the site of less but more chaotic activity; at the uppermost level is Flossy's pottery studio, and since she spends most of her time in the house, working with her pottery, it is reasonable that the studio be the acme.

A short stairwell topped by a skylight leads to a warm, richly decorated hallway. At one end of the hall is a bathroom, shower, and washroom area. A pleasing, slightly inclined bridge at the other end leads to the master bedroom. The bedroom is a retreat, and the bed is positioned to view the outline of the almost biblical sandstone cliffs against the night sky.

Energy conservation is realized through design. The house is heavily insulated, and the windows near sitting areas are composed of thermopane glass. All windows except the one facing east are tinted to cut down on solar incidence (the setting sun reflects off the ocean, causing some overheating problems). Shade overhangs would be very useful, though coastal fog tends to screen the sun to some degree. Most of the windows are in the south walls; there is a minimum of glass on the windward north and west sides.

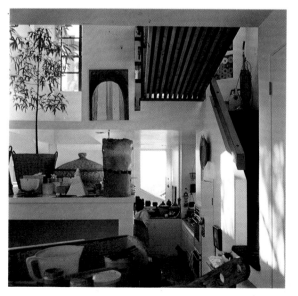

47

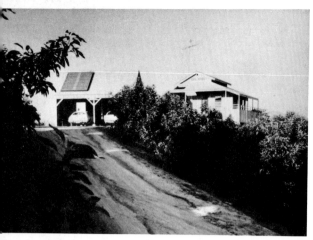

Andy is building the solar heating system himself. The collector panels are on the garage and would have been more effective if a building height limit had not prevented a higher-angle orientation. The 48 square meters (525 square feet) of copper-tube/copper-fin collector panels will heat water that will be stored in a 1250-gallon steel storage tank buried next to the garage. A single-loop heat exchanger from the storage tank to the house will provide an estimated 75 percent of home and domestic hot-water heating. Fin-tube radiators installed in the floor will convey heat throughout the house. A $\frac{1}{12}$-horsepower pump will pump water through the house and a $\frac{1}{6}$-horsepower pump will move water from the storage tank through the collectors. Andy feels that this active system should meet most of their heating needs with little trouble.

Rob Quigley's philosophy of building a house to fit the people is reaffirmed in a very different home in northern San Diego County. The people who live there have retired to an 11-acre avocado grove, in the center of which, perched on a small hill, is the house. The owners are elderly and lead a quiet life in this rural setting.

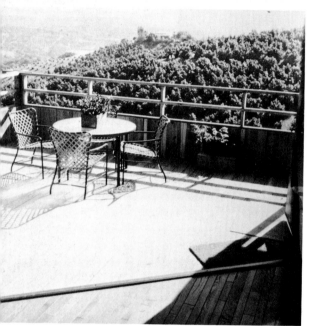

The 177-square-meter (1900-square-foot) farmhouse is a passive house, with an active system for heating domestic hot water. The design parameters for the farmhouse are less limiting than those for some other Quigley projects, and by manipulating natural advantages, the architect has achieved a thermal steady state.

Many of the passive solar benefits are derived from using traditional California farmhouse design features. The veranda and deck are oriented for the most beneficial shade and sun. The deck, like that in the Saunderses' house (page 23), acts as a solar collector. The roof color is light for maximum reflectivity and cooling. Again, there is only a limited amount of glass on the north and west sides of the building, but the south and east sides are quite open. There is a fireplace in the living room, which is completely insulated on the outside.

People who live on the top of a mountain have to be concerned about the wind. An earth berm on the northern side of the house deflects harsh winds over and away from the house, yet the wind is also used for cooling. The center of the house is raised sixty centimeters (2 feet) above grade. Cool air from this crawl space is vented into the house at kitchen and living-room vents (this principle is similar to that of the old "coolers" farm folk once had in their kitchens). The whole house acts as the cooler: as air in the house warms, it rises via a natural stack effect to a huge, central, high-ceilinged room and escapes through clerestory windows. The kitchen is centrally located in this room, and appliance heat is disposed of through the clerestory windows.

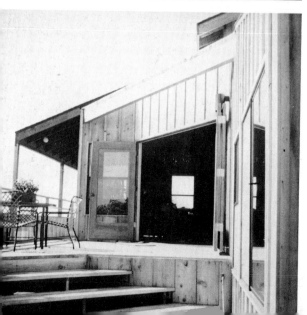

The hot-water system was manufactured by Jack Schultz of San Diego. Locating the collectors on the garage roof means they can be optimally oriented without having to worry about house orientation. This solar water heater, like so many others shown in this book, uses a heat exchanger and has a backup electric system. The complete unit, including installation, cost $1600.

48

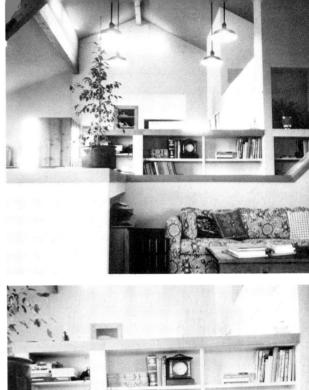

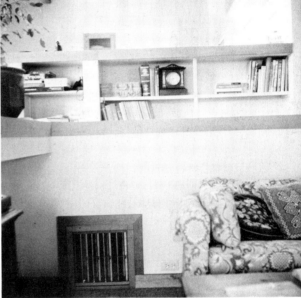

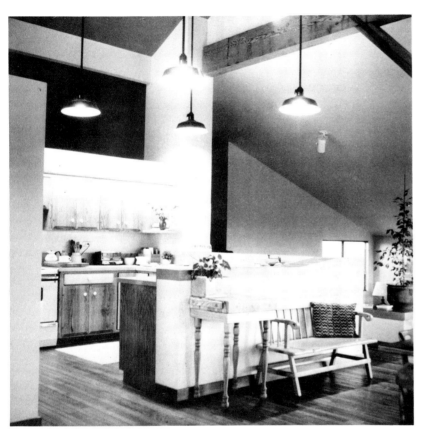

As an architect, Rob feels he is a generalist and that his goals are holistic. He is trying to create not the perfect solar house, but rather the best possible mental and physical living environment.

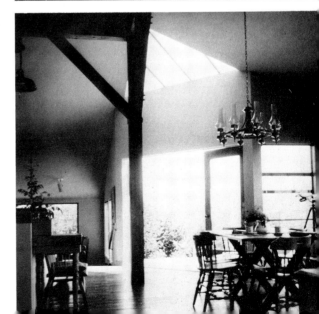

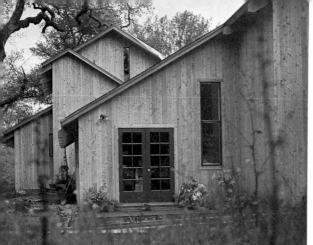

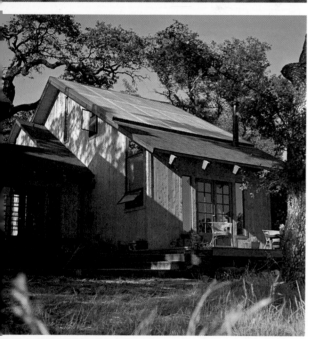

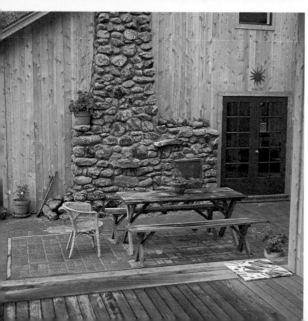

Interactive Resources

Marilyn Goode's solar home is nestled in the foothills of California's north-coast wine country. Even without the solar applications, the house is most interesting. The setting is made to order—a small stream is conveniently situated only steps away from the back door. Gnarled, spreading oak trees frame the house, and a front-yard carpet of colorful wild flowers serves as a perfect welcome mat.

This house was designed by Interactive Resources, Inc., an architectural group in Point Richmond, California. This organization is currently working on more than thirty solar projects, including ten homes in various stages of completion. According to the group's president, Tom Butt, IRI is designing houses that integrate all phases of energy conservation, esthetics, and cost effectiveness. IRI is giving clients a comprehensive service by first educating them in the need for energy conservation, and then, together with the client, designing and implementing structures that will best meet predefined goals. The Goode home was designed with these criteria in mind.

The 167-square-meter (1800-square-foot) house was first properly insulated and then provided with both space and water heating, compliments of the sun. The system is a dual one. One portion of the collector panels—3.7 square meters (40 square feet) —is covered with Filon. Water heated in these panels passes through a three-way valve into a 328-liter (82-gallon) storage tank. The mixing valve is necessary because summertime water temperatures can be expected to reach 82° C. (180° F.).

The second system designed for space heating is a forced-air system that is thermostatically controlled at two points in the house. This thermostatic control gives Ms. Goode the option of heating the entire house, the living room only, or just the sleeping area. It's as simple as operating any conventional central heating system. The basis for solar application here is 33 square meters (360 square feet) of collector panels that heat water and store it in an insulated 6000-liter (1500-gallon) septic tank stored underground. The one glaring mistake made in this aspect of the system was the failure to place the roofing under the collector panels. On the first of our two visits, the collector panels were leaking and had to be covered with tarpaulin. Nevertheless, a substantial savings will be enjoyed if 75 percent of the annual space-heating needs are met as projected. Electric heating costs about $180 per

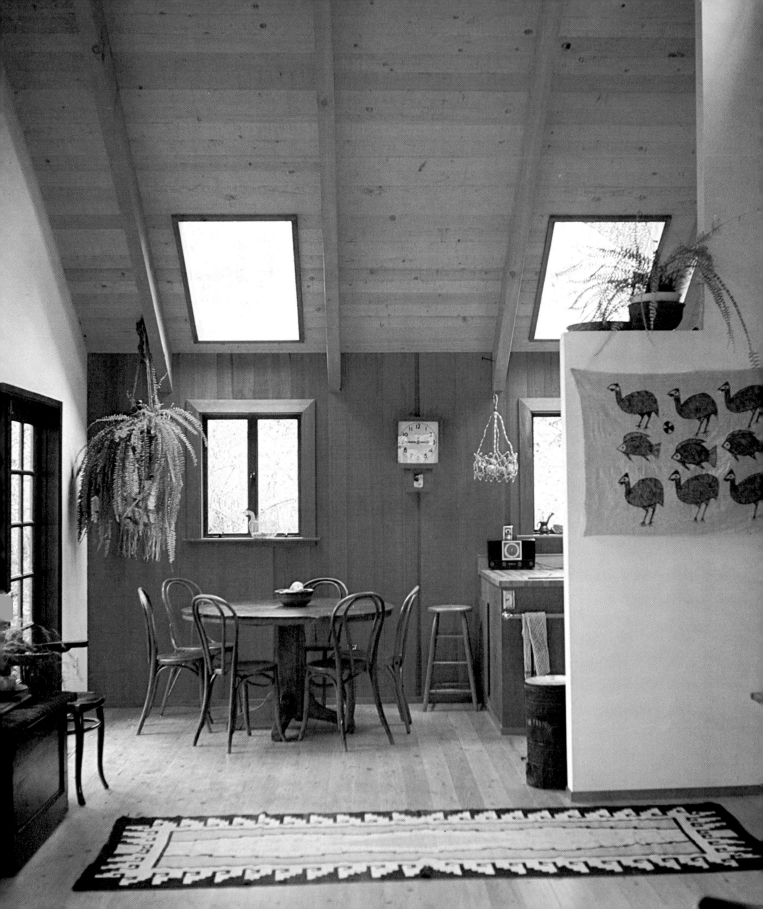

month during the coldest months of the year, while a more economical heat-pump system costs about $65 during this same period. Based on these comparisons, the solar system, which costs $7000, will pay for itself in ten to twenty years, assuming there is no marked increase in heating costs.

The house works only because it was designed with solarization, climate, and site in mind. Perhaps these total energy applications will be fostered by public utilities like Pacific Gas and Electric, which is monitoring the performance of the Goode house to determine if solar energy is feasible in the area.

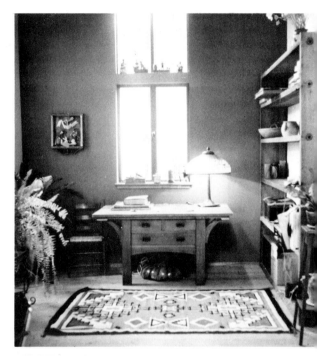

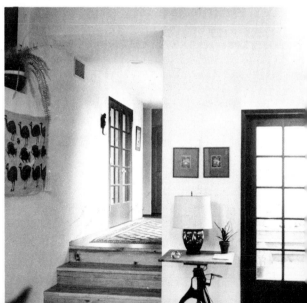

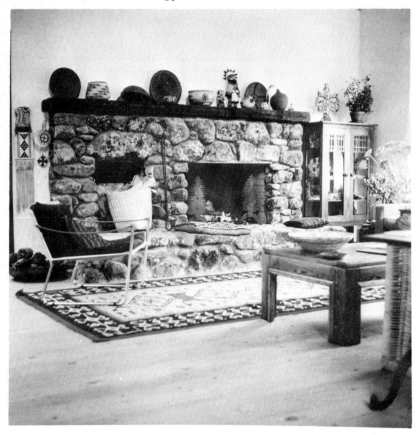

Urban Homesteading

New York City, "The Big Apple," inspires visions of the Empire State Building, Fifth Avenue, Madison Square Garden, and an endless list of people, places, and things. Seldom does the tourist (or the middle-class New Yorker) care to confront Harlem, the Bowery, the South Bronx, or the Lower East Side. Yet one of the most moving experiences we had while researching this book occurred in a five-story tenement located at 519 East 11th Street between Avenues A and B in Manhattan's Lower East Side. A brief history of this building—that is, of the people who live here—will illustrate the significance of what is now happening.

The seventy-five-year-old building is typical of the structures one finds in this area. Before October 1974, living conditions in the building were abominable. Though the landlord was neither paying taxes nor providing utility services, he was collecting exorbitant rents. Furthermore, the rooms were small and crowded, forcing families to live in half-rooms and in the hallways. In an attempt to retaliate, the tenants organized a rent strike, but in a few months fourteen mysterious fires gutted the building. Litter and dehabilitated cars, left by car strippers, prevented the city fire trucks from getting to the address. Even the tenants sometimes failed to call for fire department assistance, considering it useless.

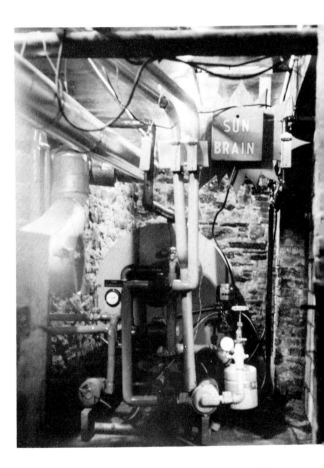

Normally, buildings such as these are vacated and taken over by the city after three years. Sometimes the city will try to administer a tenement but more often the building is demolished. Worst of all, these dilapidated buildings have a debilitating effect on the neighborhood.

In the case of 519, the former tenants, with assistance from people like Travis Price and Michael Freedberg, decided to take over the building. An almost unbelievable municipal loan of $177,000 (a mortgage) was granted by the city. This loan provided the cash to buy materials and pay the now shareholder-tenants $3 per hour in a sweat-equity program. At this writing, eleven enlarged apartments and two community store fronts are in various stages of completion.

The real story in this project, as well as three other projects in the area that are in the process of being renovated, is the human one. However, in the case of 519, people's interest in material wares has made the hardware the number-one attraction. Travis Price, who previously worked with a solar partnership in New Mexico, Sun Mountain Design, is the energy coordinator for the

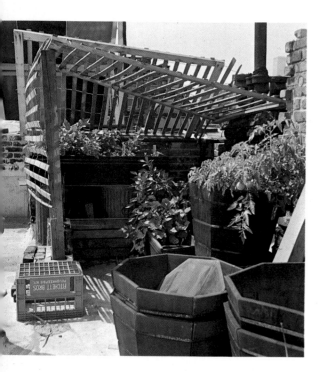

renovation. Thanks to his efforts, a $43,000 federal grant was made through the Community Services Administration to finance energy conservation and alternative energy applications in this project. About 85 percent of hot-water needs will be met by the 55-square-meter (600-square-foot) set of flat-plate collectors. These collectors are made of copper fin and tube, and the copper absorber plate was painted with a highly selective absorptive black coating. The collector panels installed on the roof of the building at a 42-degree inclination add a subdued dimension to the New York skyline. The glazing is nonreflective tempered glass. A 2200-liter (550-gallon) hot-water storage tank with a heat exchanger is located in the basement. A conventional water heater provides the backup system. Price estimates indicate that the hot-water costs per room will average twenty-five cents each month; at these rates the $11,000 system will be amortized in less than six years.

A 2-kilowatt Jacobs wind generator has been installed on 519's rooftop. Taking advantage of New York's favorable winds, this wind electric system will provide about 99 percent of the common electrical needs of the building.

More cost effective and important to the residents' comfort is the insulation that is being used. The Styrofoam insulation and storm windows will reduce heating costs by 55 percent. Passive energy conservation and the 20 percent reduction in heating needs achieved by solar-generated hot water may determine whether or not the co-op tenants will be able to pay off their mortgage loan. One estimate is that the money saved on water and space heating will amount to $4000 per year. Over a thirty-year period, the length of the loan, these savings will total $120,000—more than 70 percent of the entire construction loan. All figures are conservatively based on today's energy costs.

The changes occurring on East 11th Street are not piecemeal, and eventually they will involve the entire community. The people of the area will gradually become their own landlords and help themselves to help others. Already there is a small rooftop garden at 519. This garden will serve as the seed for a more comprehensive food-growing program. Vacant lots (lots where other tenements have already been razed) will be cleared and organized into minifarms. Closed-system aquaculture will provide a year-round protein supplement. Solar installing and insulating companies based on the 11th Street project will provide self-help opportunities for the economic development of the community.

The ultimate plan is to establish an integrated community—one that has helped itself to a more equitable social, political, and economic status. The key to achieving this status is in creating opportunities for people to apply their own toil cooperatively, because it is only through grass-roots efforts that all neighborhood residents will be able to free themselves from the state of dependency in which they are now trapped. Technology is the minor input that will insure the long-term economic success of this basically human revolution.

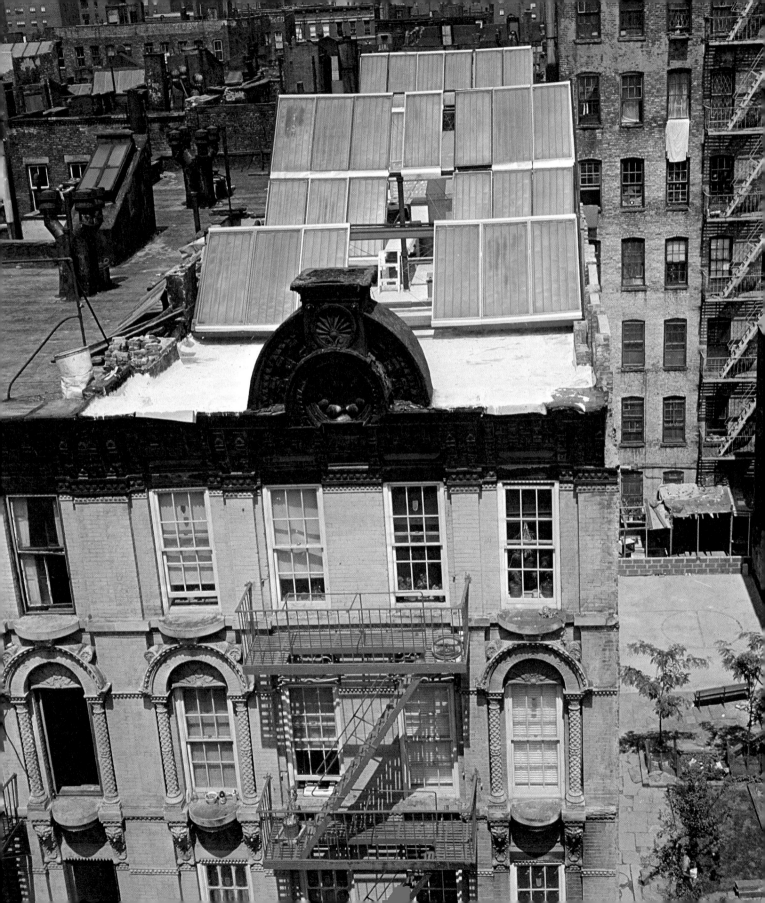

The Crowther/Solar Group

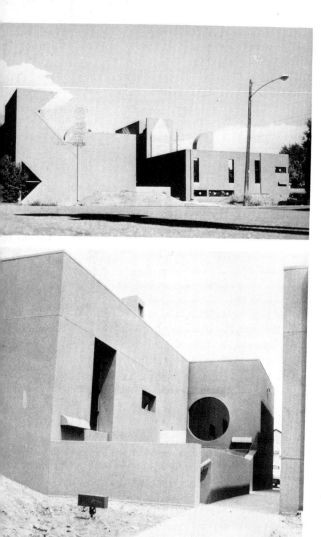

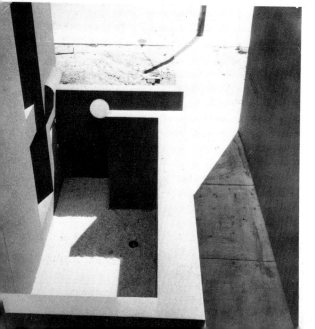

There are two new buildings in the Cherry Creek section of Denver that are clearly different from neighboring structures. Designed by Richard Crowther of the Crowther/Solar Group, they are the ultimate in energy conservation for commercial office buildings. One of the buildings, pictured here, serves as the Crowther/Solar Group's new headquarters. A total design approach—including site orientation, natural ventilation and lighting, solar heating, abundant insulation, internal building air circulation, shading, appropriate use of glass, and other applications—will make the two buildings 75 to 80 percent solar-heated and 60 percent solar-cooled.

Richard Crowther approaches architecture as an ever-evolving science. No two of his buildings are identical because no two building uses, family life-styles, or sites are exactly the same. The result is a building style that attempts to meet individual human needs, while conserving energy and complementing the environment. In architectural jargon this is *comprehensive architecture.*

The New Crowther/Solar Group building, one of the twenty energy-conserving projects that Crowther is presently composing after more than forty years of architectural research and planning, is a model of what commercial buildings should be. The 418.5-square-meter (4500-square-foot) structure combines passive and active solar systems with a tightness that keeps heat loss as low as 12.1 BTUs/hour/square foot, whereas other similarly sized commercial complexes lose ten times that amount through their glass alone. This building is heavily insulated for the severe Colorado climate: both ceilings and walls have a resistance factor of 45. Thermopane windows and tightly sealed joints further reduce air leakage.

Commercial buildings usually have fewer heat requirements because lights and human bodies create heat in confined spaces. In many such buildings air conditioning is necessary even during cold weather. By using task-lighting schemes and natural illumination, Mr. Crowther has materially reduced the heat produced by the banks of lights to which we are so accustomed. The building's total glass area is less than 10 percent of the floor space, but thoughtful planning provided both illumination and visual openness. To further illustrate the detail of design, the unusually shaped windows also play a role in illumination and space.

The windows are covered with a special reflective surface that reduces the penetration of incident summer sunlight to 22 percent, compared to more than 80 percent of light and heat that gets through normal glass. All windows are double-glazed for further reduction of warm- and cool-air loss—anywhere from 38 to 59 percent in comparison to a single pane of glass. Some windows, especially those on the south, are recessed, allowing the warmth-giving winter sun entry but shading the building's interior from the hot summer sun.

Tightly sealed joints, doors, and windows are equally important in reducing infiltration losses. Mr. Crowther designed his new office with uninterrupted insulation from the foundation base to the top of the roof. Added to this is a 6-mil plio-film continuous vapor barrier, another example of passive-energy conservation. To optimize energy performance, the office is set 4 feet into grade. These berms serve to direct the prevailing winds away from the building's surface.

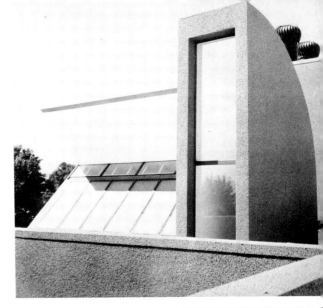

When warm air reaches the highest point in the building, it is either vented by a wind-powered roof turbine or it ventilates the solar collector before being vented. In the evening or late afternoon the ground-level vents draw cool air into the building to replace this vented warm air. On the outside the vent hoods prevent direct wind flow. Inside there is an insulated door with a gasket to prevent infiltration when they are closed. If the outside temperature is too hot to allow natural ventilation, heat pumps are used to remove the warm exterior air. Auxiliary heating is also provided by these heat pumps.

When the building is being heated, the hot air that rises is returned to the lowest level of the building. However, before this air is reintroduced into the heating system, it is cleaned by fiber, charcoal, and electro-static filters. This recycled air is usually cleaner than the outside Denver air and doesn't require the BTUs that the cooler outside air would.

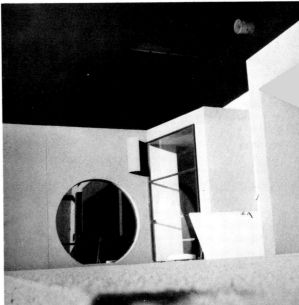

The solar collectors are the product of the Solaron Corporation, also of Denver. These air-type collectors cover 16.26 square meters (175 square feet) of a 45-degree south-facing bank. A rock storage system serves as the medium in which heat is stored. These collectors are estimated to provide 15 percent of the building's total heat requirements. At the top of the collector is a skylight that meets a reflecting-mica overhang. This stucco-mica-coated mirror reflects winter sun directly through the skylight for illumination and gains in direct heating to the north side of the building. In the summertime the overhang shades the skylight. The flat portion of the roof is covered with a white quartz-marble rock. The low-angled winter sun reflects diffuse radiation into the collector for a 15 percent increase in efficiency. In the summer, when the sun is almost directly overhead, much of this radiation is reflected back to the sky, thus reducing the cooling requirements of the building.

There is also a sun scoop over the entryway for lighting and winter solar gains. The north building, Mr. Crowther's office, has a greenhouse and a negative ion exchange unit. This isn't all, but it should suggest what Richard Crowther was able to engineer into an ordinary office building. A visit to the Crowther/Solar Group would enable you to experience commercial building architecture firsthand and see their continuing Institute for Energy Concepts display.

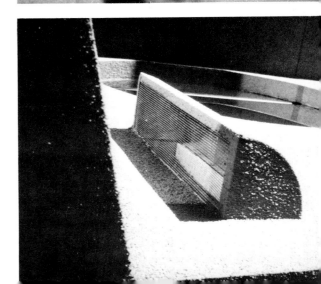

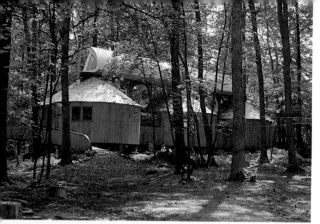

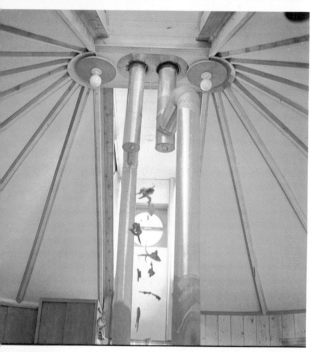

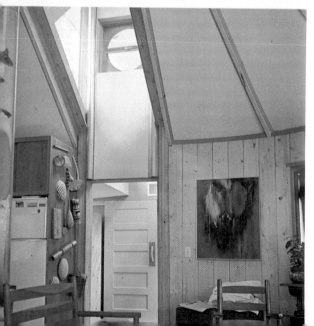

Two Swifts in a Silo

The 1973 energy crisis marked the beginning of an inflationary period from which we have still not recovered. Housing costs have escalated so rapidly that people have turned to housing alternatives in an attempt to meet one of the basic human needs: shelter.

Charlie and Mary Lou Swift live in three silos hidden in a forest near the New Jersey–Delaware border. Though it's true that these structures were manufactured by the Unadilla Silo Company near Coopertown, New York, their resemblance to fodder-storage places for cattle ends there. The shape of Charlie and Mary Lou's home is more like that of the African hut. The Swifts have emphasized this resemblance by adorning the interior with African artifacts. The 6.7-meter (22-foot) diameter conical buildings are tied together by a 24-meter (80-foot) air-type solar collector. The collector occupies 37 square meters (400 square feet) and is flanked above and below by aluminum-covered reflectors that direct additional radiation onto the collector. The heated air flows upward through the collector and is drawn across and down by a fan into a 16-cubic-meter (560-cubic-foot) bin of fist-sized stones located under the middle silo. Fans drive air back to the collector or into the rooms. All fans are thermostatically controlled to give each module the necessary versatility for heat conservation.

The house is conveniently divided into three living modules of approximately 37 square meters (400 square feet) each. The bedrooms and bathrooms are located in the east module. A short hallway joins each silo, but they can be made independent of each other with the insertion of sliding doors. Above the hallways is an open clerestory that gives excellent natural lighting to much of the building. A wood cookstove and wood heater provide backup heat for the living area, and another wood stove does the same for the work area. In addition, all three silos are heavily insulated with urethane foam and have thermopane Andersen windows.

The Swifts are living close to nature. Their 1.6-hectare (4-acre) lot is dense with vegetation and trees. These trees furnish adequate summertime shading to keep the house cool. They are also the backup fuel source. The use of two renewable energy sources, the sun and the trees, enables the Swifts to live that much closer to nature.

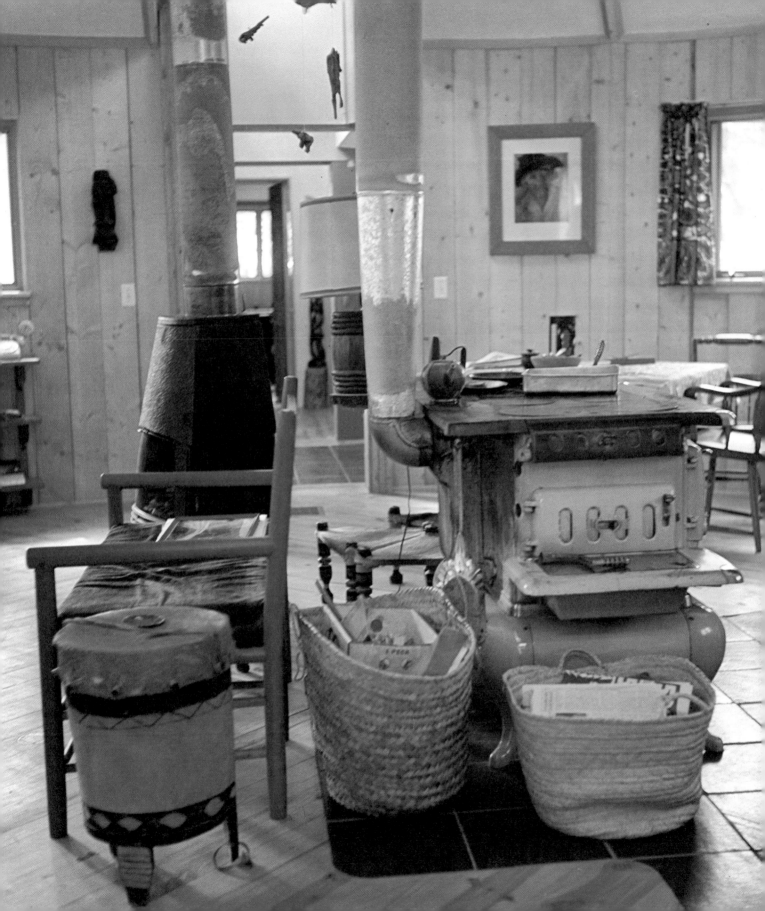

A Blueprint for Builders

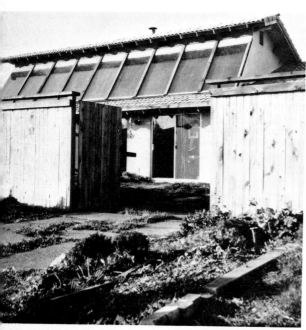

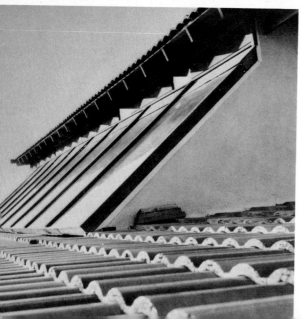

Davis is an agricultural community situated on an expanse of broad alluvial fans in the heart of California's Sacramento Valley. The city may be politically unique in the United States: it has an energy-saving building code. Led by Jon Hammond (see page 18) and Marshall Hunt of Living Systems, Loren Neubauer of the University of California at Davis, and many others, a movement was formed for the adoption of this retrofitted building code. Basically, it requires that new homes constructed within the city limits implement cost-effective energy-saving design features.

The adoption of the building code by the city council didn't just happen. A great deal of time and energy was spent in insuring its approval. A preliminary plan called "A Strategy for Energy Conservation" was presented to the council. The proposal was holistic, dealing with solar rights, neighborhood layout, street sizing, vegetation, as well as the home itself. Mike Corbett, an environmental developer, produced physical evidence of the usefulness of the plan in the form of a home he built in a recently developed suburban neighborhood. This home, owned by Chuck and Janice Ward, was the first of its kind in the community. It looks like most other houses on the block, except for the nine 1.2- × 1.8-meter (4- × 6-foot) windowlike panels discreetly designed into a dormer on the roof. Then, of course, having the right people on the council and doing a vigorous, plausible selling job were necessary to get final community commitment.

The Ward house has a passive-active system that meets 75 percent of the hot-water and space-heating needs. Actually, the solar-tempered design of the house takes care of more than 50 percent of the heating and 88 percent of the cooling needs, and the solar system accounted for the remainder. The 19 square meters (216 square feet) of collector panels heat water that flows via the thermosiphon principle to an 800-liter (200-gallon) well-insulated storage tank in the attic. Within this storage tank is a heat exchanger that heats domestic hot water. The hot-water system is tied in with a gas-fired water heater that furnishes backup heat when sunlight is insufficient. A 62-watt ($\frac{1}{12}$-horsepower) pump circulates water from the top of the storage tank into a 238-meter (780-foot) array of copper tubes embedded in a 15 centimeters (6 inches) thick concrete slab that forms the floor of the house. The arrangement behaves just like a conventional radiant-heat system, with thermostats controlling the flow of water according to water and room temperature.

The 112-square-meter (1200-square-foot) house has 16 square meters (175 square feet) of vertical south-facing windows that provide gains in direct heating and also heat the concrete-slab floor. These windows were manually covered with decorated Styrofoam panels 2.5 centimeters (1 inch) thick to prevent excessive heat loss. The Wards have a Franklin stove and a gas wall furnace for auxiliary heating. During the mild winter of 1975–76 the pilot light on the gas furnace was never lit.

Cooling costs in California's semiarid central valley are greater than heating costs. Daytime temperatures hover around 35° C. (95° F.) but plummet to 13° C. (55° F.) at night (a south-to-north sea breeze from San Francisco Bay accounts for this temperature drop). The relative humidity averages a low 30 percent. Venting the house to the night breezes causes the slab floor and other heat sinks to cool during the evening. High daytime temperatures were tempered by shading the house, using light-reflective exterior colors and heavy insulation of the whole structure, and providing enough heat-storage capacity to absorb interior heat.

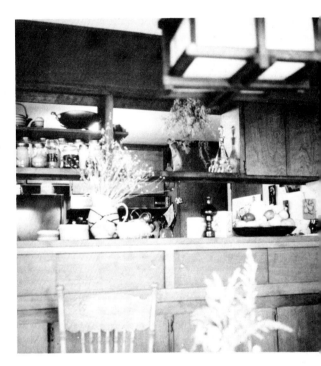

This house and lot cost $32,500 in 1974. The solarwares contributed $3500 to that cost. Utility bills in Davis have not been particularly high; at the present annual average of about $330 (including all appliances), it will probably take more than fifteen years for the energy-saving costs to pay for the additional solar costs. On the basis of economics, therefore, most people in this area would not be inclined to solarize their homes. However, fuel shortages and inflationary prices for energy should encourage them to think twice about using the sun. The quiet comfort and dependability of solar energy, plus the freedom from commercial energy sources, may be worth a great deal.

Village Homes is a 200-home development by Mike Corbett. The houses here are being constructed according to the ideas already described, and the tract also has a minimum of asphalt and a maximum of vegetation to make for cooler summer temperatures and more pleasant surroundings. We've included this unfinished Corbett home to show some of the simple yet very effective energy ideas that should be used in new subdivisions.

Each side of this "common wall" house, or duplex, measures 106 square meters (1150 square feet). The common wall is soundproofed with 15 centimeters (6 inches) of insulation. Each duplex rests on a concrete slab, and the eaves of the roof project to shade the bank of south-facing thermopane windows. There are few windows on the north and west sides, to reduce heat loss and late afternoon overheating. Exterior walls are two-by-six studs on 60-centimeter (24-inch) centers for R19 insulation. The ceiling will be insulated to R25. The tile roof is light in color to reflect the intense summer sun. These tiles are self-ventilating: they have a continuous front-to-rear air space through which air can move upward and out as it is heated. One duplex is outfitted with a thermosiphon water-heating system similar to the one in the Ward home. Cor-

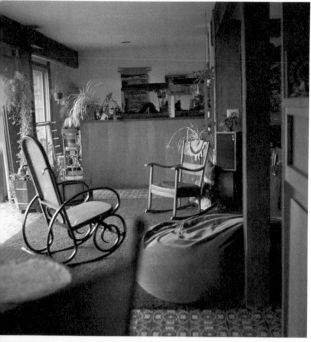

bett's domestic hot-water heaters cost an additional $700. Mike said that he is having trouble convincing people of their long-range cost effectiveness. Most people have opted for the conventional heating system.

Village Homes is a planned energy-conserving development. Outdoor space use is being planned to maximize its functionality for the homeowner. This is especially important for homes that are built on prime agricultural land, since as much of this soil should be preserved as possible. Another consideration is to assure all homeowners of the efficient use of the sun. Houses must be properly oriented to give maximum heat gains and minimum losses. In planning a neighborhood street layout, lot size and shape, and the size, shape, and height of buildings and vegetation, must be integrated in order to gain significant solar benefits. Landscaping is an especially important tool for moderating the valley's hot summer temperatures. Large deciduous trees will shade buildings, asphalt, and concrete during the summer but allow the sun through in winter. I personally feel that vegetation should be selected for its shading ability and tolerance to drought conditions. In this rather dry climate native plants would probably be best. The plans described are not utopian, but they would certainly make any community a more pleasing place in which to live.

Davis's new building plan is hardly a harsh and austere program infringing on the individual's life-style. On the contrary, the plan shows how substantial energy savings can be enjoyed simply by planning a community so that people can live well with much less energy.

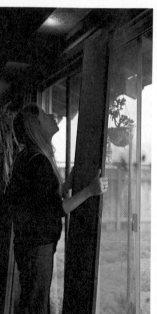

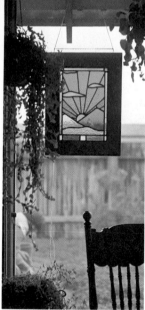

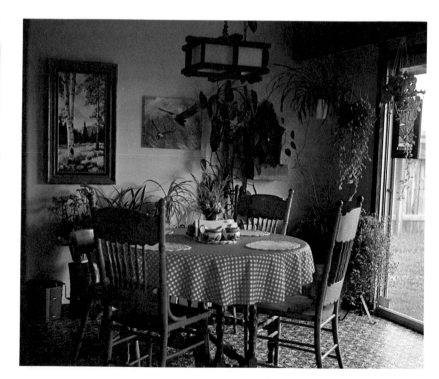

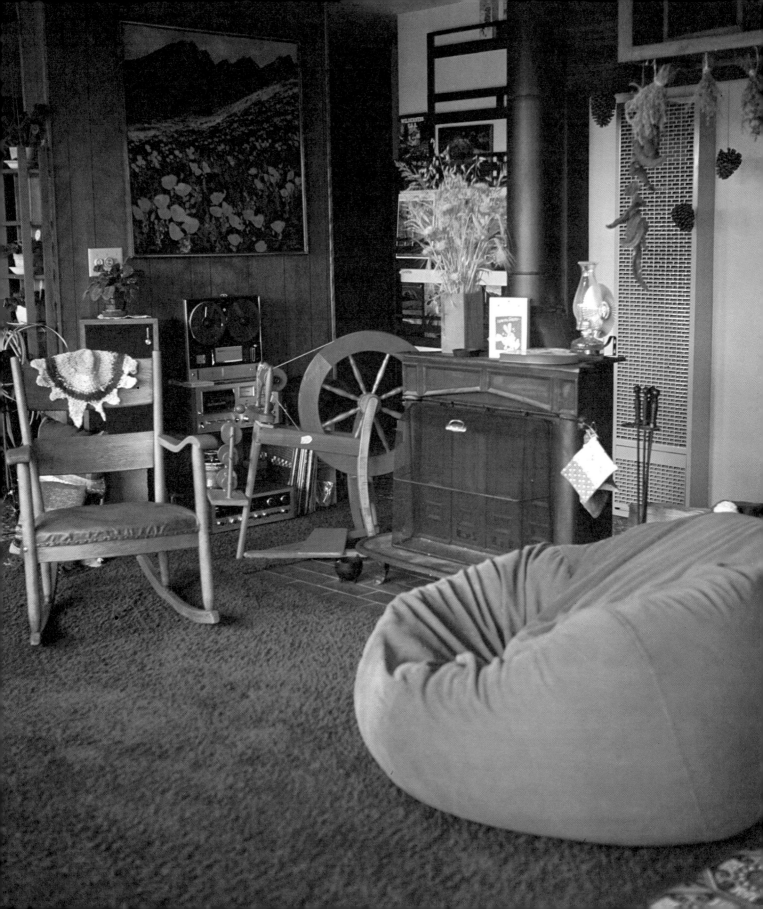

Corson's Holistic Truncation

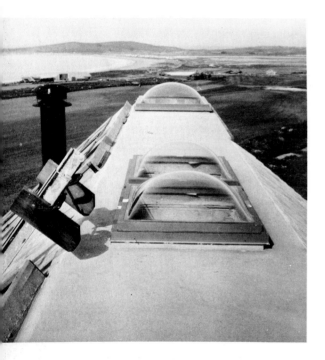

The harsh weather of California's northern coast would seem to make this area an unlikely place for a solar house. On the contrary, when the weather is bad and energy costs are high, any available economically-priced resource should be used. Undaunted by coastal fog and prevailing sea breezes, designer Bruce Corson has designed and built an energy-conserving home that is a blend of some old, established East Coast ideas with new applications of alternative resources. Bruce, who in 1974 completed graduate work in architecture at the University of California at Berkeley, built the house with several friends. Theoretical modeling predicts that this house will meet about 75 percent of the hot-water and space-heating needs through solar energy collection. (Solar projects are much more effective if the house is designed with the climate in mind.) Basic passive design features that would make any house more comfortable include: caulking of all exterior joints, wall and ceiling insulation that exceeds code requirements, thermopane glass on all windows, large southerly-oriented windows, and a reduction in window area on the north- and east-facing sides of the house.

The only unusual aspect of this house, owned by a University of California professor, is the truncated roof. The chopped-off portion of the roof is necessary because the other portion is mounted with a series of flat-plate collectors, angled at 42 degrees. This angle is ideal for catching the winter sun that heats the water that flows through the collectors. If the roof had been completed as a gabled roof, the building-height code for the area would have been violated. The truncation was a law-abiding compromise that has added character to this solar home. The skylights provide additional natural lighting.

This 150-square-meter (1600-square-foot) house is already providing numerous benefits to the owners—views of the Pacific Ocean, a pleasant blend of openness and private space, an interior that will improve as the redwood ages, and of course, the knowledge that valuable natural resources are being conserved. Furthermore, the house is esthetically pleasing because the sun-bathed colors of the interior foretell the rich warmth one experiences upon entering.

The collector system comprises seven panels totaling 30 square meters (330 square feet). The panels are two galvanized

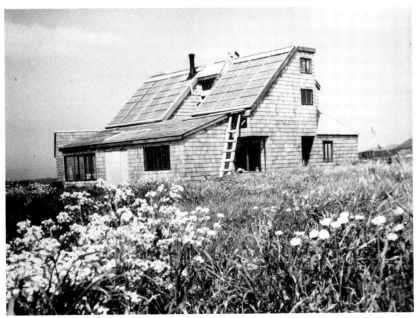

steel sheets bolted together with edge gaskets. Rubber grommets between the sheets seal the holes through which the bolts pass. These collectors have been glazed with glasteel Tedlar-coated fiberglass. Water is pumped through the panels by a super little Danish pump called a Grundfos. Because the system is a low-pressure closed loop, pumping is tremendously energy efficient. The pump draws a maximum of 0.85 amps at heads from 1 to 4 meters and flows of 5 cubic meters per hour (4.5 to 22 gallons per minute). The water in the system is stored in an insulated 4000-liter (1000-gallon) tank located in a small basement under the house. The design of the water-storage tank is practical: because this reinforced concrete structure is part of the house, its thermal mass provides additional passive heating benefits. Solar-heated water from the storage tank is pumped through copper pipes looped under the brick floor of the first floor. Here a typical hot-water radiant-heating system carries atypically heated water. Upstairs, fin-tube baseboard convectors carry solar-heated water to complete the space-heating system.

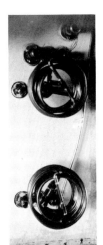
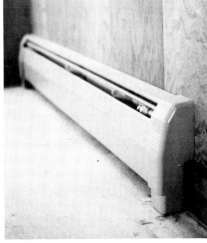

The flooring of the bottom level deserves special note because it is much more practical than most "buried" radiant systems. A vapor barrier between the ground and 15 centimeters (6 inches) of gravel prevents moisture from intruding into the subfloor. Five centimeters (2 inches) of a sand and cement combination through which the copper hot-water pipes pass rest on top of the gravel base. Red brick is laid without grouting on top of all these layers. After grinding, sealing, and waxing, the floor is smooth, easy to maintain, and the polished brick perfectly complements the interior redwood finish. The brick also doubles as a passive heat sink: it is warmed by the sun that shines through the south-facing windows.

The heat-exchange systems will meet year-round domestic hot-water needs. One exchange system is between the solar-

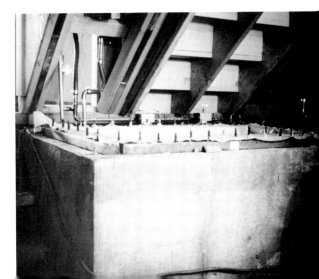

65

heated hot-water tank and the domestic hot-water heater. A back-up to the solar system, which will function primarily during times of low storage temperature, is an exchange of heat between the Franklin stove and the hot-water heater. It is unlikely that these will fail, but if worse comes to worst, a conventional electric water heater will complete the water-heating job.

The entrance to the house is common to New England but innovative for the West Coast. A front-entrance tool shed deflects the ever-present cold north wind away from the door and over the house. In addition, the entrance foyer, which is not heated, is an airlock transition zone between the cold outside and the warm inside.

Bruce has pioneered alternative energy systems on the north coast in a most original yet practical way. With a true understanding of the climate and the potential building site, almost any location can be made to work.

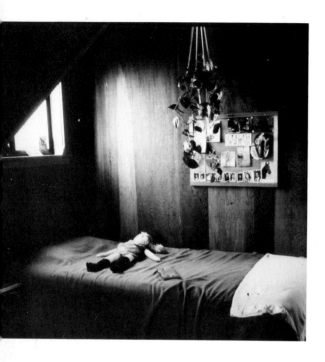

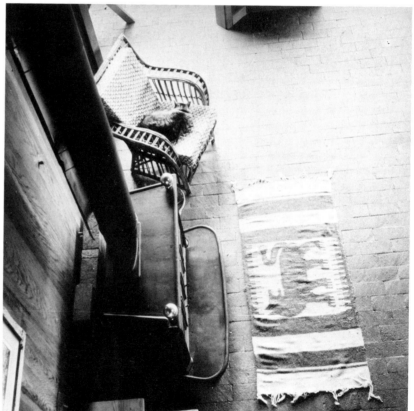

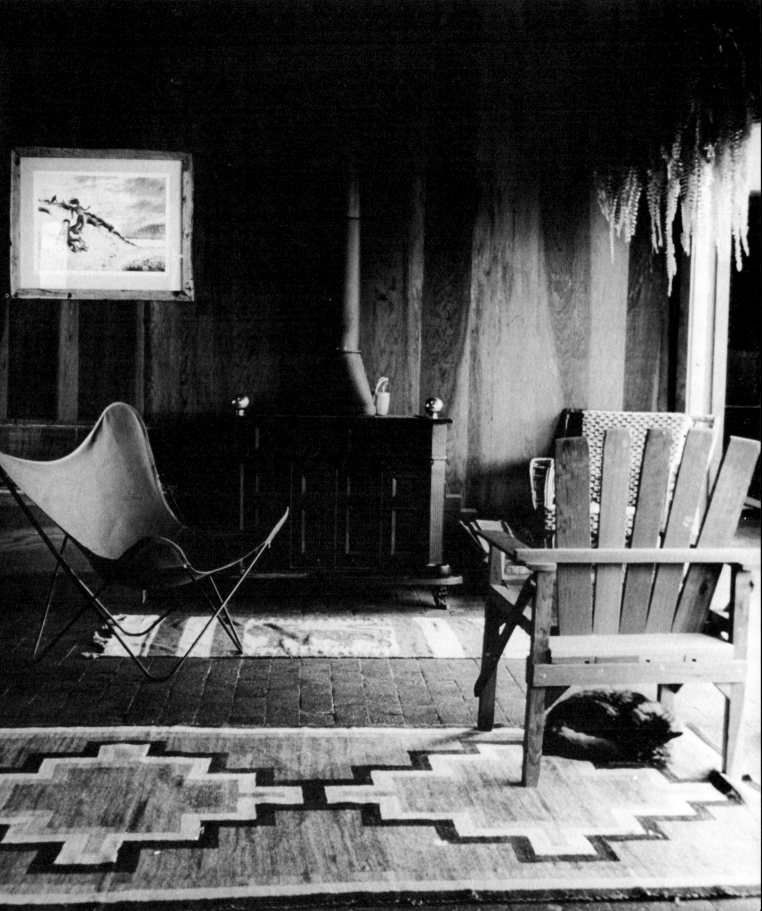

An Oregon Solar Affair

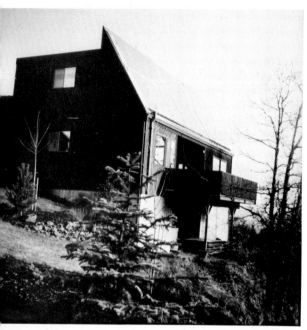

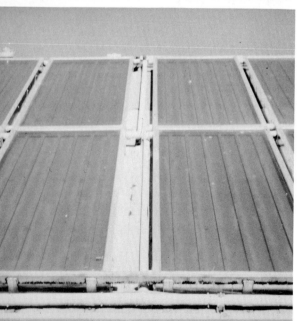

Most of the solar homes described in this book are located in areas of the United States that annually receive between 2500 and 3500 hours of sunshine. Two locations, northern New England—particularly northern Maine, New Hampshire, and Vermont—and a coastal strip that stretches northward from southern Oregon to Vancouver, British Columbia, average only 2000 hours of sunshine annually. This small amount of sun has made these areas somewhat less favorable as solar sites.

Though temperatures in the Pacific Northwest are not severe in winter, the months of December and January are bathed in sunshine only about 20 percent of the time. Nonetheless, in 1974 the Douglas Boleyns decided to build a solar home near Portland, Oregon. Foolhardy? On the contrary, during the first year of operation the dollar and cents saving for space- and water-heating amounted to $211, approximately one-third of the usual energy expenditure.

Doug and Emily Boleyn had their 186-square-meter (2000-square-foot) home built to accommodate a solar heating system. The house was designed so that the collector system, attractively integrated into the house design, would be equal to about 20 percent of the total floor space. The collectors are small because the house is well insulated and tightly constructed, thus reducing the rate of air exchange. The collectors are angled at 60 degrees, because the winter sun is low in the horizon at this 45½-degree north latitude. This relationship makes the collectors more efficient during the most crucial heat-collecting time of the year. Shading and reducing the area of glass on the west side are not as important in blocking out the hot summer sun as they would be in areas farther south.

A year after the house was built, Portland General Electric decided to sponsor the system and use the Boleyns' home as a solar demonstration project. Today they even sponsor Doug, who is energy management consultant for this public utility company that is beginning to respond with more appropriate energy uses.

The 40 square meters (430 square feet) of Revere copper panels, and the equipment that has been installed with these collectors, make this system expensive. In addition, there are many apparatuses and monitoring devices not normally needed in most homes. Generally, an active system similar to this one costs $6000 to $10,000 installed, and $3000 to $8000 if you do it yourself. These figures will be reduced as off-the-shelf items become more popular.

To heat, a 30-percent glycol and water solution is pumped through a closed-loop collector bank. A water-to-water heat exchange in the basement transfers heat to a water-storage system. Differential thermostats control the two pumps between the collectors and heat exchanger, and the storage tanks and heat exchanger. The pumps are turned on when there is a temperature difference of about 11° C. (20° F.) between storage and collector. Water is stored in three 5000-liter (1250-gallon) insulated fiberglass tanks. The total storage capacity will provide about five days of heat storage when charged to 67° C. (120° F.) at an average ambient temperature of 4° C. (40° F.). A fan-coil unit then distributes heat to the house through a duct system, either directly from the collectors, from the solar storage tanks, or from an off-peak-power storage tank, should the former two fail to meet heating needs.

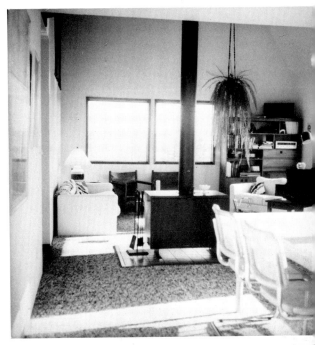

At this time, off-peak power seems more important to public utilities than to the general public, but before long everyone will realize that prime power time is an important consideration as the demand for power exceeds the utility companies' capability to meet it. Peak power use across the country varies, but generally greatest power demands occur in the morning before work and in the early evening about mealtime. If energy could be used at times other than peak demand, it would greatly reduce strains on the generating capabilities of some public utilities. In the case of the Boleyn home, a 24-kilowatt electric boiler heats a fourth storage tank, the backup system, during off-peak hours. Portland General Electric hopes to demonstrate that solar heating can help a utility shave peak demand, and to show how more inexpensive off-peak energy can be used as backup heating to a solar system.

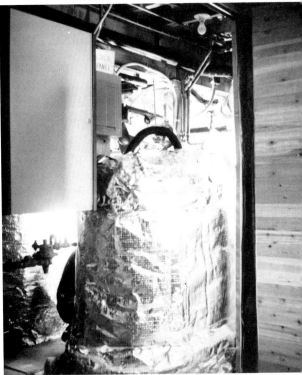

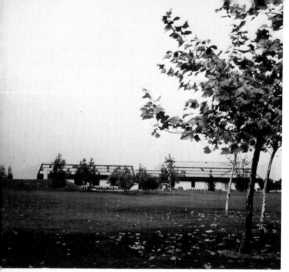

Santa Clara's Sun Project: The Community Recreation Center

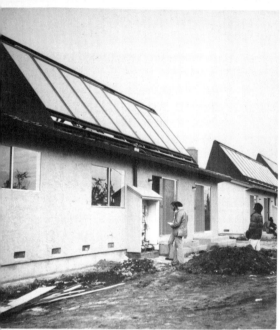

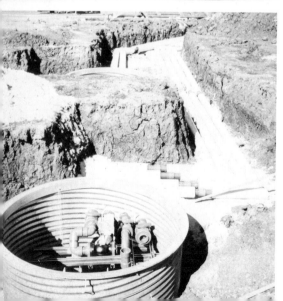

At one time, the fertile valley of Santa Clara, California, looked to the sun to dry its fruit. Solar energy is once again in use, but this time its beneficiaries are the people whose homes occupy the site of the former orchards.

The city of Santa Clara offers its residents electricity, water, and sewage services, and is now involved in various facets of solar heating and cooling in order to determine how solar energy systems might best be used as part of the public utility operation. The Community Recreation Center, which is jointly funded by the National Science Foundation, the American Public Power Association, and the city of Santa Clara, is the largest solar installation we visited. Approximately $600,000 is being invested in the 2500-square-meter (27,000-square-foot) building. Forty percent of that money will go toward the solar system. (Air conditioning has been a major contributor to this high cost.)

Originally, the center was not designed with solar applications in mind. The long axis of the building runs east and west, so the panels—650 square meters (7000 square feet) of Olin Roll Bond aluminum—were positioned on the south-facing cortin steel roof. The cortin steel enables one to work on the roof with little chance of damaging it and is also resistant to possible water damage from leaky panels. In the summer the panels heat water to about 105° C. (220° F.). This heat is used in conjunction with an Arkla Li Br absorption chiller for air conditioning. When heat is needed, solar-heated water is pumped from the panels to a set of coils across which air is blown by a fan.

A 40,000-liter (10,000 gallon) underground foam-insulated water storage tank stores hot water for use when the sun doesn't shine. This tank should provide three days' worth of carryover during cloudy periods. Another similarly constructed tank of 200,000 liters (50,000 gallons) contains chilled water to be used for air conditioning. It is predicted that these two arrangements will provide 84 percent of the heating and hot-water requirements and 65 percent of the cooling needs. Of the total energy needs, it is expected that 75 or 80 percent will be provided by the solar system.

A twelve-month study to evaluate the operation of the system was begun in late 1976. This study is expected to provide a realistic projection of the system's costs so that Santa Clara and other municipal and public utilities can properly evaluate the applicability of solar heating and cooling.

In the meantime, Santa Clara is promoting solar installations in private homes in the form of swimming-pool heaters. As of November 1976, twenty-six solar swimming-pool heaters had been installed. Fafco panels, costing about $35 per square meter ($3.25 per square foot), reduce gas costs about 40 percent during colder weather and are the heart of these pool heaters. The city charges $200 for the pool-heating installation. Then a bimonthly utility charge of $30 is levied. In the name of conservation, Santa Clara would like to convert all gas pool-heating systems to solar.

Santa Clara is also involved in a cooperative project with the federal Housing and Urban Development. A HUD grant has been received to build six homes with heating systems similar to the one used in the recreation center. These homes will be conventional looking and will be monitored to determine what approaches should be taken in the future.

Cities like Santa Clara and Davis are setting patterns that other communities could well study and modify to fit their own climates and social situations.

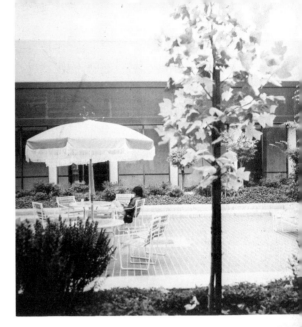

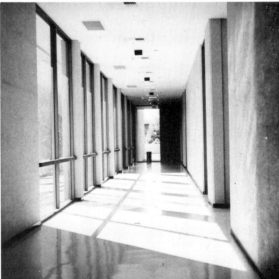

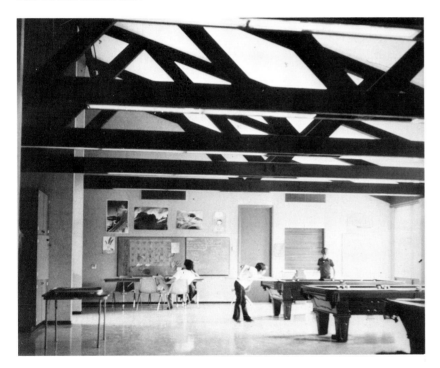

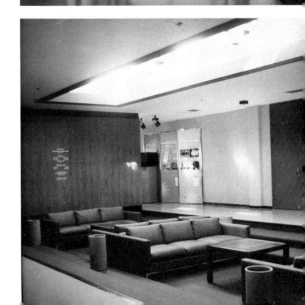

Rocky Mountain Sunshine

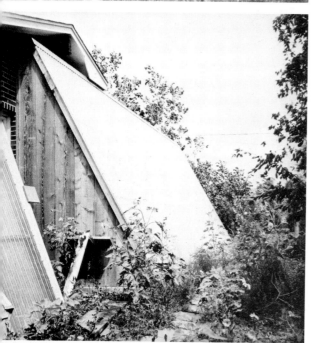

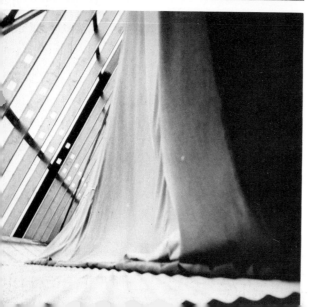

Most students of solar energy quickly realize that proper orientation toward the sun is necessary to capture its radiant energy. What, for instance, should be done in order to heat a house whose long axis runs north and south? There are a number of possible solutions, one of which, shown here, was developed by professional engineer Robert Bushnell of Boulder, Colorado.

Bob Bushnell's solar retrofit uses a detached, free-standing collector on the south end of his 186-square-meter (2000-square-foot) home. The appearance of the house has been altered, and the 3.7- × 8.5-meter (12- × 28-foot) collector adds a bit of architecture to the Bushnell backyard garden.

The collector rests on a concrete foundation and is externally covered from top to bottom with a corrugated Tedlar-coated fiberglass material called Filon. Under the Filon is a layer of glass. This whole array is tilted at 62 degrees. Behind the two layers of glazing is a large bolt of black cotton-polyester cloth. This sun-absorbing surface starts 10 centimeters (4 inches) in from the top of the panels and hangs straight down. The sides and back of the collector are enclosed by heavy insulation. Peak temperatures in this air system are amazingly high. Air in the collector was 88° C. (190° F.) the day we visited, and Mr. Bushnell said that the maximum temperature he has noted was 122° C. (252° F.).

The system works by blowing the sun-heated air into a storage bin in the basement, adjacent to the west end of the collector. The absorber cloth allows the air to pass through it and a 560-watt (¾-horsepower) blower blows the air into a bin filled with brick, concrete, and water in steel drums. Forced-air circulation across the rocks meets 36 percent of the house-heating needs. Mr. Bushnell pointed out that the system would work at about 75 percent efficiency if the house were more tightly insulated. (Sometimes it's difficult to insulate older homes adequately.)

Mr. Bushnell has been the consulting solar engineer on a number of homes in the Boulder area. One just completed, an unusually-shaped 165-square-meter (2000-square-foot) home nestled at the base of the Colorado Rockies, was designed by Earth Dynamics of Boulder. The two-story house combines passive and active solar applications. The shape of the house made it possible to engineer passive design features. The prevailing north winds are directed over the top of the structure by the low-inclined north roof. The bottom floor is protected from winds by an earth berm.

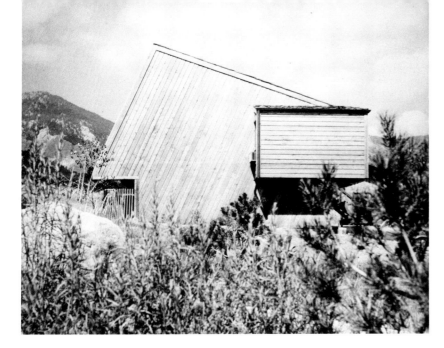

Most of the windows are located on the south side, but there are west windows to permit gains in direct heat in the bedroom in the evening, and north windows for the view.

The second-story sunporch adds another dimension. Not only is there a fantastic view of the Rockies, but the enclosed area is warmed by the sun in the winter and cooled in the summer by the shading stemming from the protruding collector panels. Behind the sunporch a bank of collector windows provides gains in direct heating. The picture shows the summer shading imparted to these windows by the collector panel overhang.

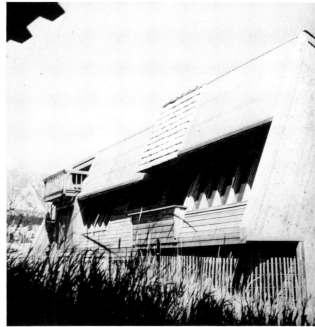

Twenty-four square meters (256 square feet) of Filon-covered collectors heat air for storage in a 7200-kilogram (8-ton) rock storage bin located between the laundry room and the bedroom on the bottom floor. A forced-air heater with a two-stage electric back-up system is thermostatically controlled to function when the temperatures are cool. A differential thermostat determines whether the heat is extracted from the rocks or whether electricity will have to be used. Predictions have it that about 70 to 80 percent of the winter heating needs will be met by the active-passive combination.

The Bushnell system uses air and rocks as the transfer and storage media, respectively. A rock storage system is a little less than half as effective as an equal volume of water. Therefore, in sizing the storage system to the house and designing for the maximum continuous time period without sun (a guesstimate), a rock storage system would have to be larger than a water storage system in order to do the same job. But there are advantages to using rock. One, you don't have to worry about watertight tanks and leakage with rocks (although both types of storage containers must be insulated). Two, rocks do not corrode or leave dissolved solids, as water sometimes does, nor do they freeze. If storage capacity is sized correctly, rock and water storage do the job equally well. The medium selected will depend on its availability, the design of the house, and other limiting factors.

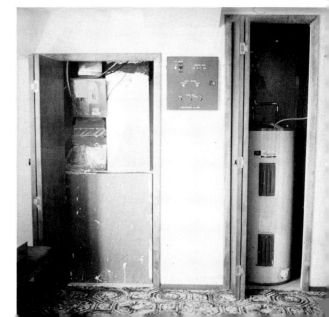

73

Solaris

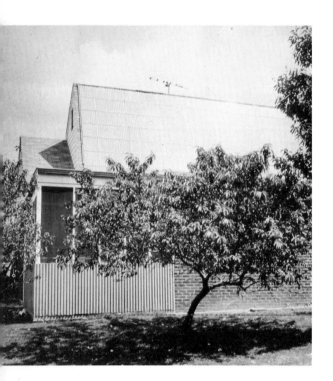

Harry E. Thomason built his first solar home in 1959. At that time, a solar-heated house was a newsworthy event, but few people were seriously interested in owning one, particularly since fuels were still relatively inexpensive.

Mr. Thomason holds more patents in solar energy than anyone else in the world. But an even more significant achievement, in this time of expensive energy and very expensive homes, is the fact that he has an off-the-shelf solar heating system that makes the cost of his houses competitive with conventionally heated homes. In the fall of 1975 a North Carolina construction firm was building Thomason-fitted solar homes for $37,000, the same price as homes with conventional heating and air conditioning. Furthermore, the Thomason collectors, marketed under the brand name Solaris, have proved to be about 75 percent efficient in converting the sun's radiant energy to heat energy stored in water.

The Thomason Solaris System is simple and straightforward —as simple as rain running off a roof. On a hot sultry day in 1956 rain from a freak thunderstorm running off a sun-heated sheet-metal roof provided the impetus for Harry Thomason's affair with solar energy. A black-painted corrugated aluminum sheet is the absorber plate. The aluminum is housed in an insulated box and covered with either one or two layers of glass. Water from a pipe along the ridge of the roof is distributed to the valleys of the sheet metal. As the water flows down the absorber plate toward a gutter at the bottom, it is heated. The heated water then flows to a storage tank under the house.

Thomason Solar House No. 3, where the family now resides, is a 255-square-meter (2750-square-foot), single-story, four-bedroom home. The garage, indoor swimming pool, and game room—a total of 139 square meters (1500 square feet)—are not heated. Approximately 89 square meters (960 square feet) of trickle-type collector panels are tilted at a 60-degree angle on the south roof. A 4.5- $\times$ 12-meter (15- $\times$ 40-foot) sundeck over the swimming pool–game room area directs additional winter radiation onto the collectors, increasing their efficiency by about 15–30 percent. The sunporch is also a passive collector; it receives both direct-gain heating and heat from the swimming-pool water during the winter.

A 10,000-liter (2500-gallon) concrete storage tank in the basement contains about 6400 liters (1600 gallons) of rainwater. Rainwater is collected from the north roof, and then filtered and delivered to this storage tank. The tank is surrounded by a 59.5-cubic-meter (2100-cubic-foot) bin, containing fist-sized stones. In the heating mode solar-energized water flows from the roof to a heat exchanger for domestic hot water, then into the storage tank. Eventually this water is pumped back to the roof for reheating. In the meantime, heat from the water is conducted to the rocks. When the house gets below a thermostated temperature, a blower turns on and draws cool air from the house, blows it across a filter and the warm rock bed, and back into the house for warming. If the rocks are not warm enough, then an auxiliary oil furnace is activated, using the same duct system.

During the night the house is cooled by an air conditioner that, in turn, cools and dries the rocks. On hot days house air is blown across these cool rocks and is then recirculated back into the living spaces. This method of cooling is much less costly than conventional methods because the air conditioner operates during off-peak demand times, the period of lowest electrical rates.

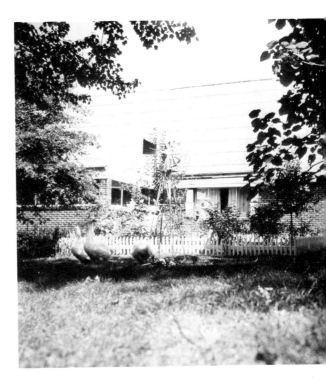

At about $43 per square meter ($4 per square foot), Mr. Thomason has probably the least expensive active solar system on the market today. The collectors are lightweight and their efficiency is as high as 80 percent. Critics say the system is overrated because water condensation on the underside of the glazing reduces efficiency. Basin-type solar stills do have much water condensation on their glass covering, but nevertheless distill water effectively. In 1959, Mr. Thomason spent $4.65 for heating oil in his first solar-heated house, versus costs of about $100 for a nonsolarized house. Something had to be working for him to save that kind of money. The USDA solar dairy experiment (page 114) is testing four different kinds of panels, including the Solaris. The results of these trials, which are being conducted near the Thomason home, should give valid data on the comparative performances of various collectors.

Energy conservation appeals to most Americans only if it is cost effective and does not require too great a change in living standards. Alternative energy applications will become more and more cost attractive as fuels become scarcer and more expensive. In the meantime, Harry Thomason is offering a product that, coupled with good housing design, should be seriously considered by anyone who can afford a new home today.

Herrington's Homespun Habitat

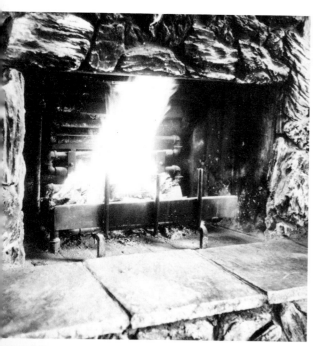

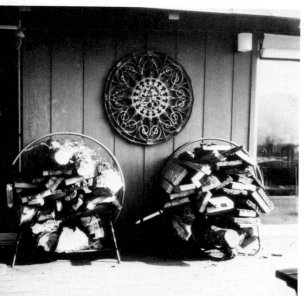

Ken Herrington's mountain retreat in Napa County, California, is a lesson in the production of home-grown energy. A professional industrial photographer, Herrington is earnestly working toward the preservation of precious fossil fuels, and is teaching others how this can be done.

Popular Science has referred to Ken as a "do-it-yourselfer." More aptly, he is a one-person research institution. His ideas are creative and practical and their effectiveness has been proved through careful monitoring and record keeping. Two major Herrington projects are a fireplace-fueled, forced-air heating system, and a solar hot-water/swimming-pool heater.

People like fireplaces in their homes for both increased heat and esthetic reasons, but in reality, most fireplaces are no more than 10 percent efficient. Ken felt that he was not getting the mileage he should out of his fireplace and came up with an inventive way of using it to benefit the entire house. The fireplace was converted into a hot-water/radiator: water is pumped through a pipe grate to be heated by the fire, and, when heated, augments the performance of the forced-air heating system. In designing a "water grate" that would be efficacious, he carefully researched and discovered the hot spots in the fireplace. This, and the fact that he was able to determine which size wood would produce the hottest fires, has reduced his heating gas costs by $150 per year, based on late 1976 prices. (The savings would be even greater today because the $150 figure was arrived at by averaging the last three years' performance, though the water grate has been improved since its installation.) Total costs for the entire hot-water heating system were $440. This cost includes an 800-liter (200-gallon) insulated hot-water storage tank that is used to heat the 204-square meter (2200-square-foot) house in the morning before the fire can effectively operate.

Ken's domestic hot-water system is completely home designed and built. The collectors, which he outlines in detail in his pamphlet *Solar Water Heaters,* are copper-tube/sheet-metal fin plates placed in insulated plywood boxes and covered with Kalwall glazing. The collectors are then plumbed into the domestic water supply via a unique heat exchanger. Rather than immerse the exchanger in the water tank, copper tubes are wound around the tank and covered with Thermon, a heat-transfer cement. Ken admits that

76

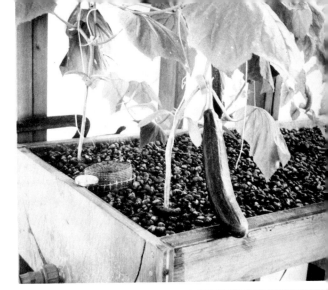

this arrangement is not as efficient as the immersion design, but it meets his needs. This hot-water system is used to heat both domestic hot water and the swimming pool.

Ken has collected some interesting data on the performance of the hot-water heater collector under varying weather conditions. On a clear February day with an ambient temperature of 13° C. (56° F.) and no wind, the collector increased storage-tank temperature by 28° C. (50° F.) The very next day, with cloudy weather and a temperature of 9° C. (49° F.), the tank temperature was increased by 22° C. (40° F.). On a clear day in early April with ambient temperature at 20° C. (68° F.) and the wind at 6.7 meters per second (15 miles per hour), the temperature increased 28° C. (50° F.). Finally, on a May day with high overcast, a 20.5° C. (69° F.) ambient temperature, and the wind at 3.6 meters per second (8 miles per hour), the tank temperature only increased 22° C. (40° F.). The point is that numerous variables influence energy gain on any given day. It seems that clouds do not cause major problems, but winds reduce the rate of temperature gain.

Ken Herrington is only getting started. He is working on a solar-heated hydroponic greenhouse. He also has plans for a more elaborate space-heating system and will eventually install a wind generator to supplement his electrical needs. The Herrington homestead is located in a natural setting, deer roam the front yard, and all domestic water comes from mountain springs. It is only natural then that the Herringtons should tap the other natural resources that Mother Nature so abundantly offers.

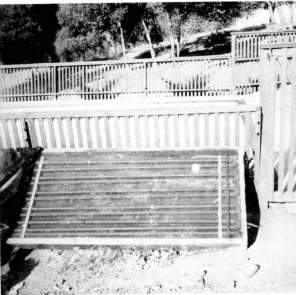

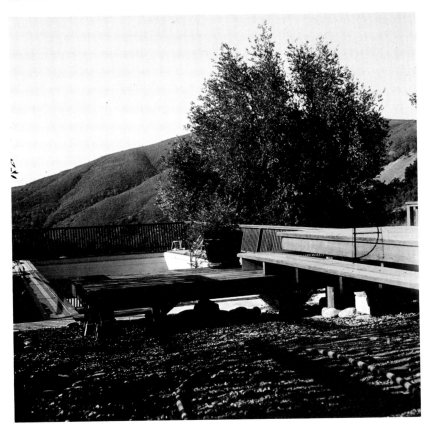

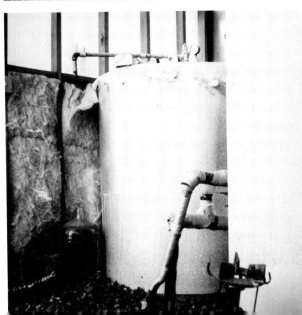

Wind-Site Evaluation

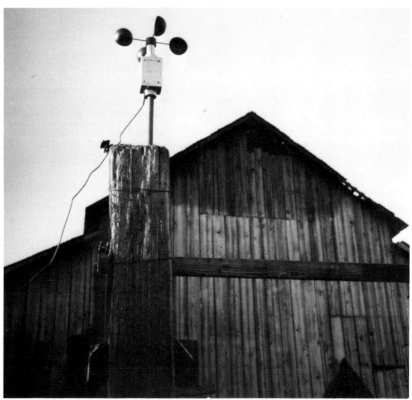

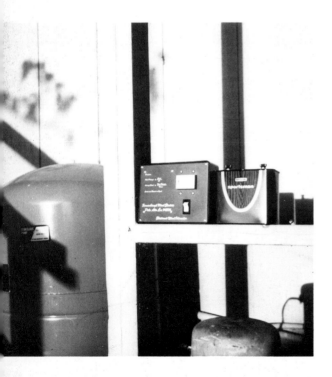

Large public utility companies and the government will undoubtedly spearhead research on wind power on a regional scale. For the individual, the benefits of wind power are many, but certain considerations must be taken into account before one thinks about installing a wind project. Site evaluation—average annual wind-speed determination and the presence of obstructions that cause turbulence—is essential.

Wind-site study does not have to be sophisticated. The Sencenbaugh wind-speed recording odometer shown here is a very accurate tool for measuring a site's wind speed. It is easy to install, and it can be read as simply as a thermometer.

Charlie's Wincharger
Downwind Airlift Jacobs Trip

The first time we met Charlie Hall, he announced that if we wanted to learn anything about wind generators, my first step should be to visit his TV repair shop in downtown Barre, Vermont. Strewn among old TVs and tubes were fat, bullet-shaped metal easings—wind generators. The morning I visited, Charlie placed a set of tools in my hand and directed me over to a 1800-watt Jacobs. The rest of the day was spent in learning by doing—overhauling the Cadillac of wind generators.

The Hall residence and workshop is surrounded by low hills and dense stands of conifers. Towering over the trees are four wind generators resting atop their towers. These generators represent Charlie Hall's first step in achieving self-reliance in energy. Eventually, three generators will furnish all electricity necessary to operate what I must call a demonstration-research center.

Visiting Charlie's workshop is like going back to the 1930s. Everything there is powered by a 32-volt bank of deep-cycle batteries that are charged by a 1600-watt airlift. His lights are 32 volt, as well as his radio, toaster, washing machine, refrigerator, and drills and grinders. An old remodeled TV set has even been converted to run on 32 volts. What's more, everything works just like our conventional 110-volt electricity.

Charlie's ultimate goal is to construct a demonstration energy-efficient, self-sufficient house. He hopes the house will serve as an example in New England of the potentialities of alternative energy applications. Of course, all electricity will be wind-powered.

In the meantime, Charlie Hall is a member of the hard-working staff at Goddard College, where he teaches a course in wind power that gives students information on everything from generator retrofitting to tower climbing. In spite of some initial apprehension, every one of Charlie's students has climbed a ninety-foot tower. His vigor in promoting wind power and greater self-reliance has had a tremendous impact on everyone who has come into contact with him. Perhaps the real Charlie Hall can be best described by his remark, "Try to get everybody to smile; it only takes seven muscles, while it takes ten muscles to frown—conserve energy."

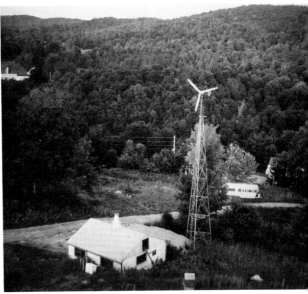

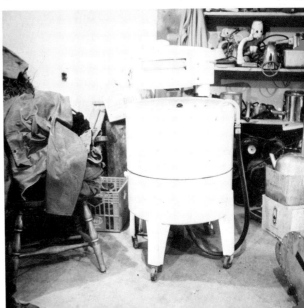

79

The 6000-Watt Electro Wind Generator

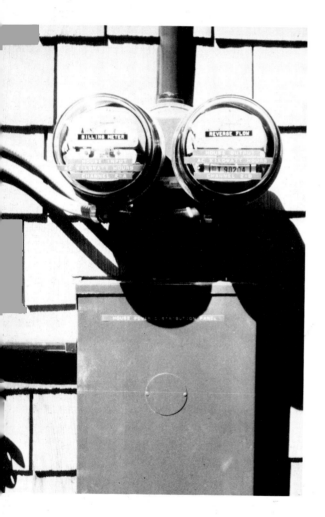

This 6000-watt Electro wind generator located in Point Richmond, California, is the world's largest commercially available electric generator. Its performance has been closely monitored by Pacific Gas and Electric. Recently purchased by San Jose State University, it will be dismantled and reassembled at the campus.

The generator has what is known as a Gemini Power Conversion Unit (one of a few in the United States and the first one of its kind in California). The Gemini eliminates the need for a storage-battery backup system for when the wind doesn't blow. The generator ties in directly with PG&E's power-grid network: when excess electricity is produced by the generator, credit is given on a typical electrical meter; when more electricity than what the generator is producing is needed, it is available from the conventional power grid and billed from another meter located next to the credit meter.

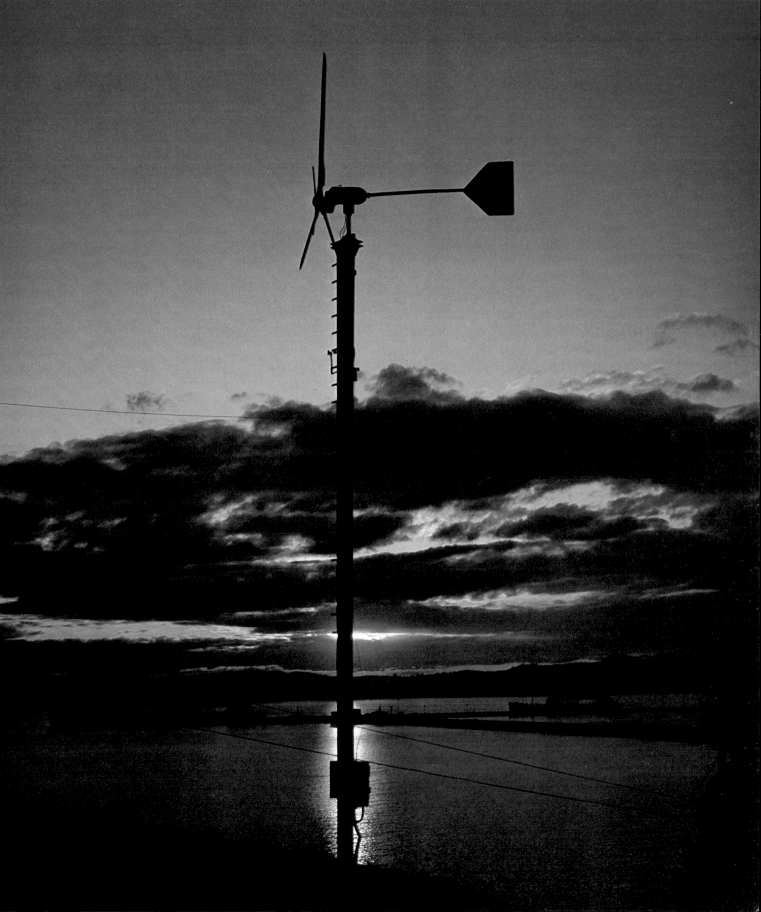

Wind Power Systems

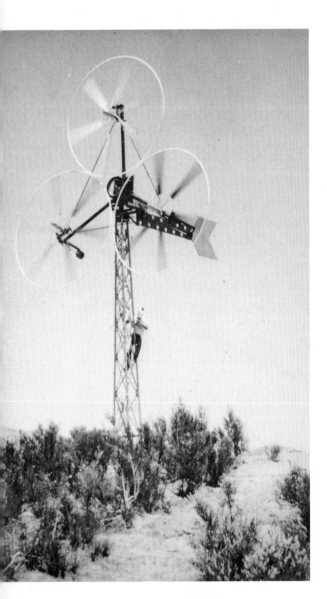

There's a new twist of the propeller in wind-power systems. Edmund Salter, president of Wind Power Systems, has put together an impressive wind generator, the RD-4000, which, at first glance, resembles three mating hula hoops. A prototype of the RD-4000 (the number means that the generator is rim driven and is capable of generating 4000 watts of electricity in a 20-mile-per-hour wind) was built and successfully tested in 1975–76. Of course, there is a difference between testing and actually operating a wind machine at a site. There are no current installations of this wind machine, but it merits mention because of numerous innovative engineering features.

The RD-4000 has three rotors that are attached to a central wheel. Each of these rotors rotates at 200 revolutions per minute, and together they drive the center wheel at 1200 rpm, thus producing the 4000 watts. One interesting safety device is the automatic feathering mechanism. The entire rotating assembly tilts as wind speed increases. This tilting action exposes a smaller surface area so that the assembly will not be blown away in a hurricane. In very strong winds the assembly is nearly horizontal, but it is nonetheless able to rotate at maximum speed and produce electricity. A hydraulic damper prevents the blade assembly from returning to a vertical position too rapidly should the wind stop suddenly. The blades on this generator are also unique. They are skinned with thin galvanized steel sheets between which liquid urethane foam is sprayed to ensure a stiffer, more durable propeller assembly.

Instead of exploiting the market potential of the tri-blade wind turbine generator himself, Ed Salter has licensed Up-Right Scaffolds of Berkeley, California, as the exclusive manufacturer. The generator is scheduled to be available sometime in 1977.

Ed has some recommendations for people considering installing a wind-electric system. One should ask oneself three general questions: (1) What kind of wind site do I have? (2) What is the price of power in my area? (3) What will be the cost of a wind apparatus that will do the job in accordance with my particular lifestyle? For example, is it really worth investing in a $600 tower, a $1500 storage system or inverter, and a $2000 generator when your monthly electric bills are $20 and your average wind speed is 2.2 meters per second (5 miles per hour)? On the other hand, in some New England states the average annual wind speed is 5.4 meters per second (12 miles per hour), and electricity costs ten

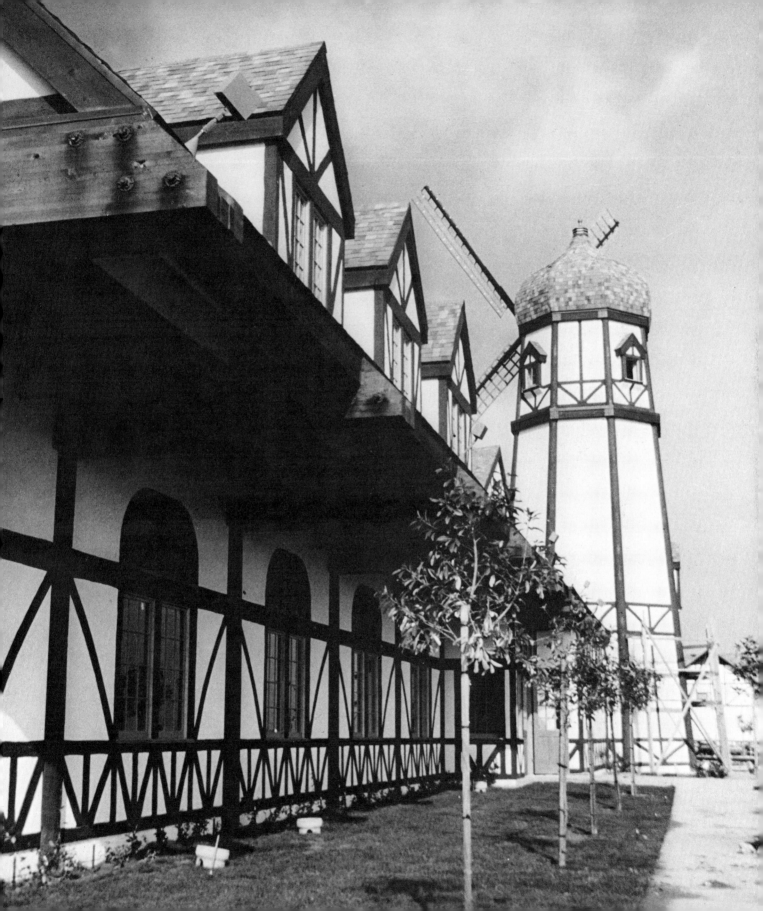

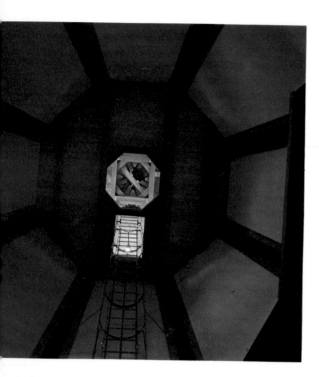

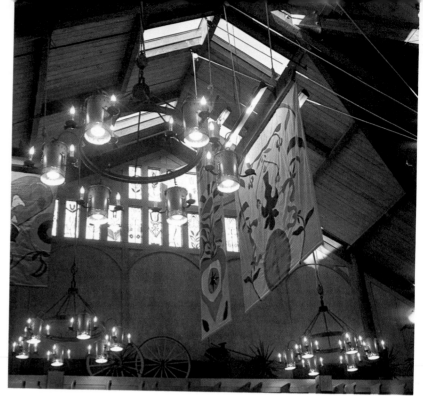

cents per kilowatt-hour. In these winds, if you have a generator large enough you could generate 1000 kilowatt-hours per month. That's $100 worth of electricity each month. A $6000 installation would be paid for in five years.

Wind Power System's latest project is a first for the United States. They were the consulting engineers and partial builders of a large Danish-type generating windmill. This replica of a European mill was engineered for Anderson's Pea Soup Restaurant at Santa Nella, California.

As you approach Santa Nella by car, you probably won't believe your eyes as they feast upon the seven-story windmill turning slowly in the late afternoon breeze. At this writing, it is the largest wind-electric system operating in the United States, and the only one of its kind in the world. (NASA's 100-kilowatt generator is having blade problems.) From outside to inside underneath the sweeping lines of the windmill cupola, the assembly is an engineering marvel. The four-bladed prop is 14 meters (46 feet) in diameter and is designed to withstand winds of 62.5 meters per second (140 miles per hour). The blades are covered with clear, shatterproof plastic sheeting 2.5 millimeters ($\frac{1}{10}$ inch) thick. The 1.1-kiloton (2500-pound) rotor combination will extract approximately 12,000 watts (16 horsepower) from a 11-meter-per-second (25-mile-per-hour) wind striking the blades head on. Blade speed appears to be very slow, but if the shaft is rotating at 25 rpm, then the speed at the tip of the prop is 27 meters per second (60 miles per hour). Since the windmill is not free to track the wind, it will be interesting to determine how much this affects the energy output over a period of time.

The rotor will turn a shaft that is geared up to 50:1. Thus, a windmill shaft speed of 20 rpm will be increased to a generator speed of 1000 rpm. Maximum generator output is about 8 kilowatts, which will be fed into a synchronous inverter. Ed Salter recommends that if you have access to the power grid, it's more practical to opt for the inverter than for storage batteries. The electricity generated is fed directly into the restaurant lighting circuit.

The windmill speed is controlled and limited to a safe 25 rpm. Should the speed of the rotor exceed this rate, a spring-activated, modified semitruck air-release brake comes into play to slow blade speed. The entire braking system is failsafe. That is, if any component fails or there is a power outage, the brake will completely stop the windmill.

Originally, mills of this type were used to grind grain, saw lumber, and pump water. The modern high-speed Stuart-type rotor is approximately twice as efficient as the four-arm sail configuration. According to Salter, the added cost of the generating system should be justified by the electricity it will produce over the next ten years. It does, in any case, serve two other purposes. First, data from this generator could pave the way for more sophisticated wind generators. Second, the entire assembly is a conspicuous display that Ed Salter feels is necessary to educate America in the resource value of wind power. Wind is a constant depositor in our energy bank account. As 50–60 percent of the land area in the United States is suitable for extracting power from the wind, wind power will become important in our quest for energy independence.

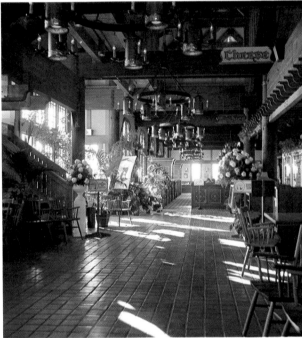

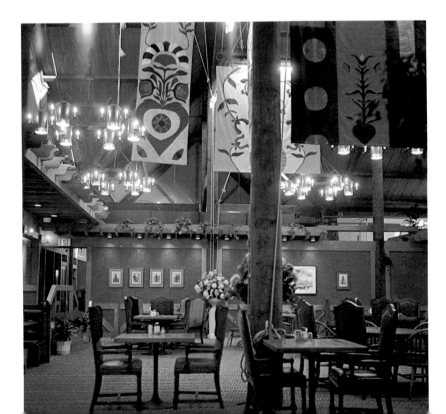

Remote Wind

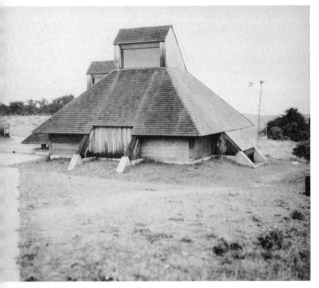

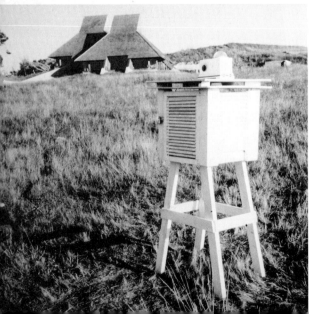

North of Sea Ranch in northern Sonoma County, California, the trees grow as if a force is constantly pulling them in one direction. There is a force, but it is pushing rather than pulling. The more vertical than horizontal sweep of the branches of these conifers is the first clue that the wind blows here both often and forcefully.

When the California State Parks Department decided to develop a visitors' recreation center at the coastal playground of Gualala, it failed to estimate what it would cost to energize the center. Pacific Gas and Electric said it could furnish electricity for an initial investment of only $20,000 for lines and poles, but the public utility services were considered unreasonably expensive for this situation. Alternatives were explored, and wind-generated electricity offered the only practical solution. But why is wind only an alternative today when it was a dominant energy force in the past?

At the turn of the century many rural and semirural areas in the United States depended upon the wind to generate electricity. The REA (Rural Electrification Administration) spelled the beginning of the end for most wind-electric generating systems. This federally operated organization forced rural folk to use public utility services whether they wanted to or not. As a result, Jacobs and Windcharger generators mounted on 90-foot towers are mostly memories of the past. The only wind application still used to any extent is the Aeromotor and its relatives, which pump water into areas too remote to be economically supplied with electricity.

The energy crisis of 1973 made people realize that our ability to produce fossil-fuel electricity will almost certainly be limited in the future. This crisis rekindled an interest in the use of wind power. At this time, however, the economical generation of electricity from wind has not been realized. With few exceptions, fossil fuels still produce electrical energy more cheaply than wind.

One of the exceptions is the remote site at Gualala. This is a special situation. Traditional energy sources were expensive because the site was off the beaten track. Since there was a high average annual wind speed, the decision was made to install a wind-electric system.

A visitors' recreation center receives most of its energy demands on weekends. The basic needs included electricity for lights, rest room exhaust fans, and the operation of a few power tools from time to time. However, the people who developed the recreation center didn't want electricity for the sake of the center. They wanted *wind-generated* electricity because they were trying to build a center that was sensitive to the environment. The design of the center made maximum use of natural lighting. There is also a water-conserving vacuum toilet in operation. The wind system seemed to fit well with their holistic ecological approach.

The generator that was decided upon was a 2000-watt Australian Quirks Dunlite mounted on a 12-meter (40-foot) tower. No on-site wind studies were conducted. However, wind-speed data from Point Arena, 24 kilometers (15 miles) to the northeast, were plugged into a computer to help make the decision on generator size. Thus far, the 2-kilowatt unit has done the job.

The alternator produces 100-volt AC current that is rectified in the generator and comes down the tower as DC. Because of current loss with DC power, the generator cannot be situated too far from the area that will use the electricity. The plant is about 45 meters (150 feet) from the building. All electrical use is DC. DC power limits the use of some appliances, a slide projector in this case, but basic needs are met. There is a bank of 19 deep-cycle storage batteries that have a storage capacity of 360 ampere-hours. Thus far, the wind-electric system has produced far more power than needed. However, there is a gas generator for backup purposes in case of emergency.

The Gualala wind generator paid for itself the day it was installed. The generator, tower, storage batteries, and installation costs totaled $6500 in 1974. What's more, this electric system means no monthly utility bills. It has been almost maintenance free.

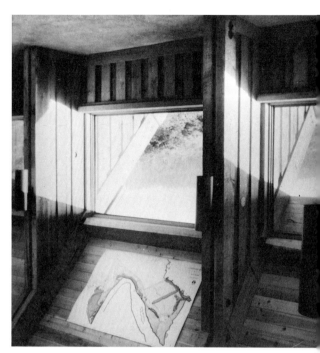

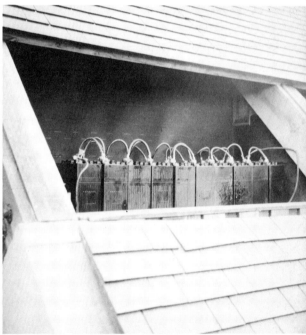

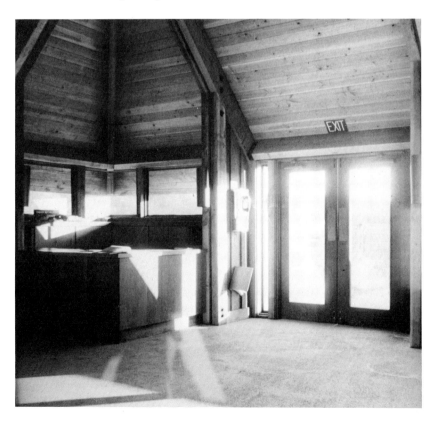

Yanda's Greenhouse Luncheon

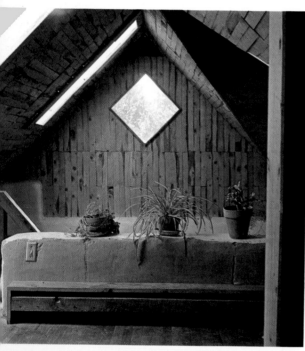

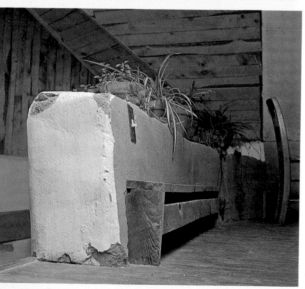

Bill Yanda has kept the design of his solar greenhouse simple. The stud framework structure, covered with a greenhouse fiberglass like Filon or Lascolite, goes a long way toward conserving energy and promoting self-reliance.

Bill pioneered the construction of solar greenhouses in New Mexico. In 1974 he received a grant from the Four Corners Regional Commission to supervise and construct eleven greenhouses aimed at helping people who live in village communities in northern New Mexico.

The greenhouses are located on the south wall of an existing home and are vented into the building through existing doors or windows or by constructing louvered vents. Not only does the greenhouse extend the summer growing season and provide year-round vegetables, but the heat can be vented directly into the house. The add-on structure, when built against adobe as in the case of Bill's house, becomes a Trombe wall with plants.

During the summer of 1976 Bill conducted greenhouse workshops throughout New Mexico. After a community was selected and materials were arranged, he demonstrated how an attached greenhouse could be erected in just two days. The first greenhouse gave the people in the community the experience necessary to build their own or to teach others.

Bill's own greenhouse was completed after he remodeled his adobe home. The seven-year-old house was purposely made to look old. A close study of the exterior walls shows the roughened adobe laced with flecks of straw. This was the style used in old adobe construction, a style that responds to the rising and setting sun with a glowing orange warmth. Although it is not considered a solar structure, the very mass resulting from the use of adobe tempers the living space against the elements. To supplement this passive feature, the house is sunk 90 centimeters (3 feet) into the ground.

Greenhouses can be integrated into the house using any material that's easily available. Bill estimates that he is building the houses for less than $21.50 per square meter ($2 per square foot). The outer glazing can be a material like Filon, and a second layer of glazing—in this case an ultraviolet-resistant polyethylene called Monsanto 602—is necessary for greater insulation. (The ultraviolet-resistant feature slows the deterioration rates of polyethylene materials caused by sunlight.) It's important that the greenhouse be airtight—leaks contribute to heat loss. Numerous variations on a heat-conserving theme can be worked out; all that is necessary is a bit of ingenuity.

Shading and ventilation must be a part of any greenhouse because even in winter the house may overheat. A partial solid roof extending over the floor space will shade plants from the high-angled summer sun. Awnings or bamboo curtains are other simple solutions to the overheating problem. A vent near the floor on the prevailing wind side and a second vent at ceiling level on the leeward side will create a natural draft and reduce heat. Ideally the downwind vent should be about twice as large as the one on the windward side. A properly designed greenhouse should not require electric fans.

Bill's greenhouses are specifically designed for use in the climate of northern New Mexico. The basic idea, however, is simple enough to be adapted to almost any climate. And adapted it should be. Solar greenhouses are energy-conserving means of extending the growing season in cold areas, and the heat can be used as supplementary space heating for the home. Finally, what better way could there be to observe the fascinating workings of Mother Nature? Considering the practical and esthetic benefits offered by these greenhouses, they may well be the most cost-effective solar application available today.

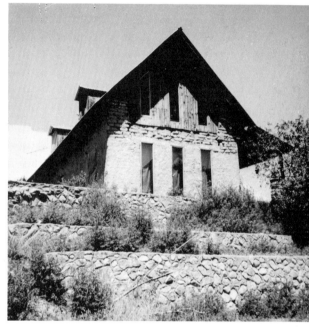

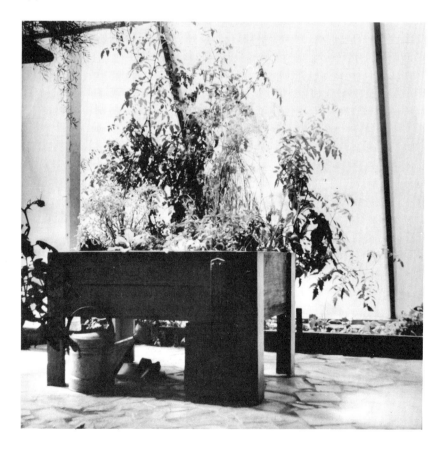

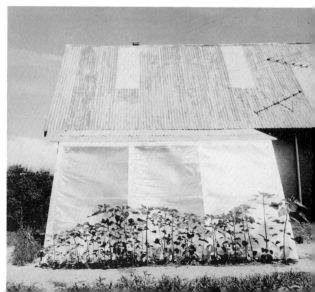

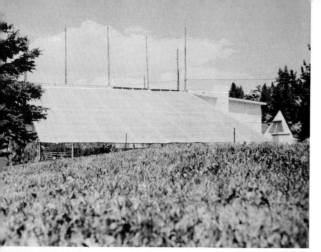

Operation Sundance

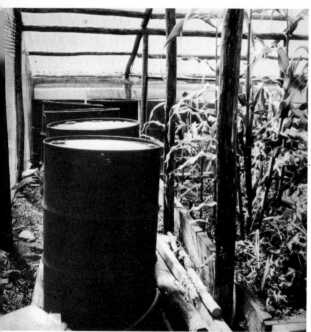

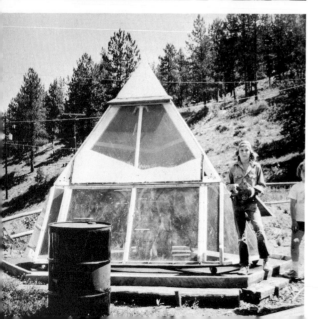

Operation Sundance, Domestic Technology Institute—a utopian fantasy? Not at all. From his headquarters in Evergreen, Colorado, Malcolm Lillywhite, director of the Domestic Technology Institute, has been the Pied Piper for numerous alternative living-system developments, including Operation Sundance.

Malcolm, a former NASA physicist, decided that helping people help themselves in their own backyards was more important than providing them with outer-space information about the weather. He has been a fountainhead of information and inspiration to people within an eight-state area. Only a few examples of his work near Evergreen are included here.

A principle we may someday revere as a "Lillywhite" is Malcolm's idea of getting people to cooperate on a community and regional basis, using indigenous raw materials and their own hard work. His idea not only results in net energy conservation, but also helps stabilize the local economy. An excellent example of this stabilization is at work in Colorado's San Luis Valley. A series of solar-energy-based workshops set up for lower-income people produced the desired self-help experiences. In addition, a few of these newly trained solar "experts" were inspired to set up small business ventures to assist others in the area.

Operation Sundance conducts courses at a public school in Evergreen under the name of The Open Living School. Malcolm is the director of this federally funded project, which is an interdisciplinary environmental teaching program for children (as well as teachers and other adults) designed to activate an interest in solar energy and other natural energy systems.

The Sundance Greenhouse shown here was totally constructed by young people between the ages of ten and fourteen. As one can see, the structural material came from the forests in the area. The greenhouse is not only beautiful, but it is also quite innovative: John Husey, one of the builders, claims that it is the first 100 percent solar-heated greenhouse with no backup system in the Evergreen area. The greenhouse will also have a large, open water-storage area—a 6000-gallon tank—that will provide the humidity for tropical plant growth. (Imagine bananas in the Rockies!) A set of scrounged radiatorlike panels will be mounted atop the structure to heat water and provide for continued crop production even when snow is on the ground. The students have also built a pyramid-shaped solar

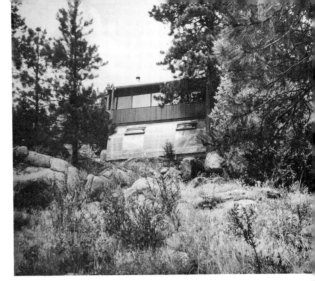

food dryer using Steve Baer's Beadwall principles. Their architectural prowess and gardening talents rival, and perhaps even surpass, those of many people in the building and farming industries.

Peter Howell is an Open Living School instructor who has gone even further in his construction of a year-round solar greenhouse. He and his wife Maggie live at the nontropical altitude of 2500 meters (8200 feet) and at a 39½-degree latitude. Their driveway is a tortuous, rock-strewn 90-meter (300-foot) path up the south slope of a mountain. Because the trail to the house is so steep, the Howells sometimes find it necessary to use a horse to carry materials to the house. Nevertheless, the view and setting are spectacular. The peaceful location is made even more habitable by the warming sun on the south-facing slope, especially in winter.

Peter and Maggie's greenhouse is constructed from a recycled army-surplus Quonset hut, the inspiration for which was the solar-energy course they took a few years ago with Malcolm Lillywhite. The greenhouse is 6 × 18 meters (20 × 60 feet) and is glazed with corrugated greenhouse fiberglass on the outside and polyethylene plastic on the inside. (An additional layer of fine-mesh linen is added for summertime shading and cooling.) To gather and store heat in the winter, 220-liter (55-gallon) black painted drums and rocks are located at various places inside the greenhouse. Windows and a door at both ends of the house are necessary for ventilation, to reduce the chance of overheating in the summer.

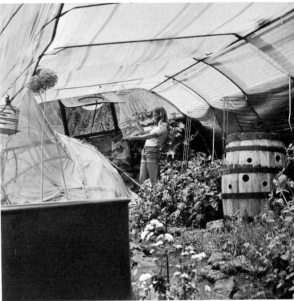

The list of fruits and vegetables that the Howells produce reads like a newspaper advertisement for a quality vegetable store—without the high prices. Lettuce, beets, and carrots are grown throughout the winter, and radishes, cabbage, peas, broccoli, strawberries, tomatoes, zucchini, onions, garlic, beans, sweet corn, cantaloupes, and herbs during the rest of the year. Thus the Howells are able to eat pretty well all year round. (Originally, the greenhouse cost about $500.)

Other projects on which Peter will continue to work include a solarized chicken coop. The chickens are an important source of eggs and meat and also provide fertilizer for the gardens. Excess fruits and vegetables are fed to the chickens. Eventually, the Howells hope to have a composting toilet, and they plan to design passive solar-heating applications into their home.

I'm sure both Malcolm and Peter must have had something to do with little John Ruskey's construction project. John is not very big yet, so it would be impractical for him to build and operate an average-sized building. Therefore, he built himself a solar greenhouse to fit his size and needs. Everything, including the 40-liter (10-gallon) black painted cans that line the south wall, is miniaturized. John's greenhouse has a couple of noteworthy wrinkles. Since the cans are so short, he places them along the south wall where they shade only a small portion of his growing space. He has insulated the north wall of the greenhouse with fiberglass batts, thus reducing winter heat loss with little loss of light available to plants.

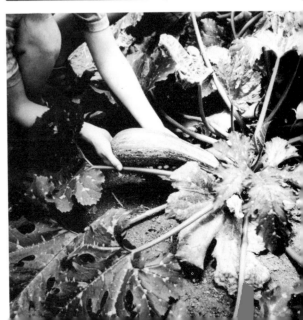

Malcolm and his right hand, Donna, collaborate on the homestead operation, which features a large solar greenhouse, an outside garden, grow holes, and a pack of Rhodesian Ridgeback hounds. As if that weren't enough, numerous workshops in alternative energy systems are conducted through the Domestic Technology Institute. Domestic technology is a systematic methodology of solving community-based problems by incorporating community-level technological solutions. Energy is the neutral focus from which a community can develop base plans to aid in solving problems and evolving a less consumptive life-style. Of course, this is only true when energy concerns are approached with the idea of using natural energies and conservation. Since what is being attacked is neutral—the energy problem—age, sex, and racial differences become less important. Perhaps if more community issues were approached in this fashion, many social problems would gradually solve themselves.

Malcolm's work is much more extensive than what has been discussed and shown here. He is one of the primary exemplars of what an individual can do in a region where people are ready to receive his expertise.

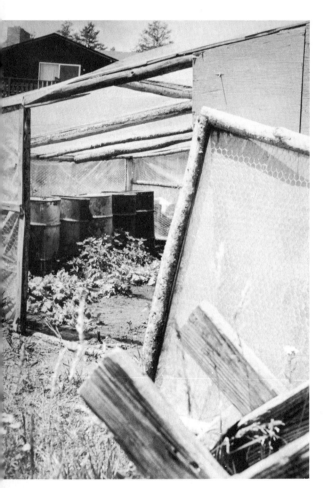

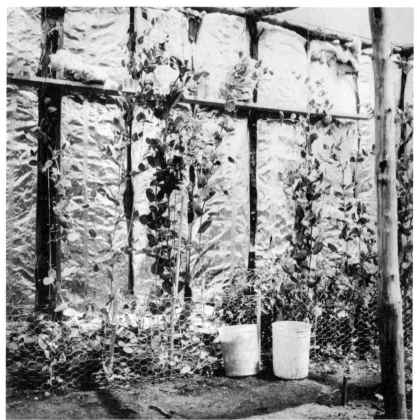

Whole Life Systems at the Farallones

The Farallones Institute of Berkeley and Occidental, California, is educating the public in energy alternatives adaptable to either urban or rural settings—all in keeping with the conceptual philosophy of the Institute, referred to as "Whole Life Systems." Whereas Americans once fled the countryside for city life, today there is a strong movement back to the land. Yet the interrelationship between city dwellers and farmers is as important as it has ever been. Under the directorship of Bill and Helga Olkowski, the Institute is trying to bridge the gaps between these two groups.

In an older section of Berkeley there is a Victorian building that bears the name Integral Urban House. Behind the façade is the Farallones Urban Center. In addition to setting an example of energy resourcefulness within the confines of a city, the people at Farallones are offering relevant courses in such things as urban food-raising, solar energy systems, aquaculture, and beekeeping.

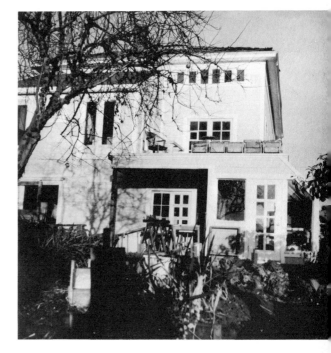

Integral Urban House has undergone quite a face-lifting—or, more appropriately in this context, a retrofitting. During the mild 1975–1976 winter rooftop solar collector panels provided the hot-water needs of the four people living in the house. Space-heating needs were partially met by an added-on greenhouse. At present, more work is being done on space heating.

Extensive research is being carried out on waste management, which the Farallones people refer to as *resource recovery.* One appliance they are testing is a composting toilet. Its biggest advantage seems to be that it uses no water, and the waste is recyclable. Our own wastes are resources that we dispose of by means of another resource—water. Our soils lack organic matter, fertilizers are becoming more expensive, and we are already experiencing water shortages. Composting toilets are very practical solutions to these problems. When the true worth of this alternative is realized, flush toilets will seem the limited alternative. The performance of the composting toilet is being carefully monitored. Eventually a gray-water management system will be installed. This water will be used to irrigate certain parts of the minifarm.

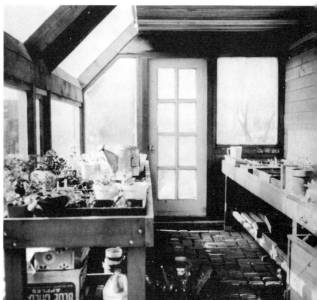

From the standpoint of size, the Farallones food production area should be called a garden, but the variety of crops grown—alfalfa, green-manure crops, and food crops—makes it more like a small farm. Alfalfa is being used as rabbit and chicken feed. Green-manure crops refurbish the biological and physical properties of the

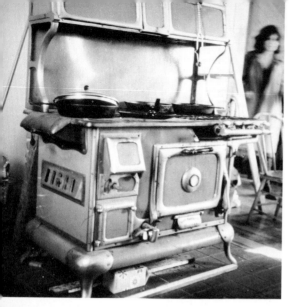

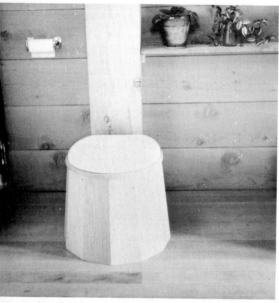

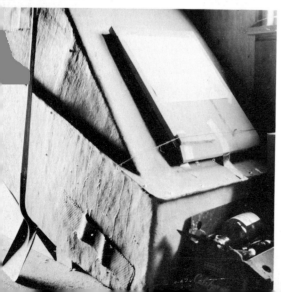

soil, and fruits and vegetables nourish people. The rabbits and chickens are fed from the garden, but they also receive table scraps and the chickens also get trapped insects. These alternative feeds do not seem to reduce the yield of meat or eggs. All refuse from the animals is added to the compost bin. The compost serves as an organic fertilizer and soil conditioner for the garden. These urban agricultural activities are closely integrated with each other and with human activities. When all facets of the urban center are considered, one begins to appreciate the whole-life-system idea.

David Katz is the manager of the Farallones rural center, an eighty-acre ranch near Occidental. Though the basic concepts are equally applicable to country and city, the scale for rural areas is much larger. Food and fiber production are being developed within a framework that is also concerned with maintaining natural ecosystems. By using a wide variety of agricultural techniques and ideas, Farallones Rural cultivates crops and raises livestock in a manner that fosters a healthy biotic community.

The human element is an integral part of this rural community. Whereas human needs tend to be met at the expense of everything else in our present ecosystem, at Farallones people's daily comforts are being taken care of in a fashion that recognizes that natural resources are finite. A "bread box" solar-heated shower provides 90 gallons of 130° F. water on sunny days. This gray-water resource is then recycled for use in the orchard and vineyard. Other solar employment is being developed to heat buildings and supply additional domestic hot water.

A sylvan compost privy furnishes the user with a private woodland view. The Farallones Rural privy is much more economical than the urban center's "clivus multrum" (a Swedish waterless composting toilet that through aerobic bacterial action changes human and vegetable wastes into usable humus). It is a vented concrete block container. The waste must be removed from its original container and put in an open bin for further composting. The decomposed feces and urine are then recycled to the soil. The rural center also has a clivus multrum. All these nutrient-recycling units are being sampled and tested for parasites and bacteria. Thus far, no human parasites or pathogenic bacteria have been isolated.

The comprehensive agricultural plan includes a .4-hectare (1-acre) garden of terraced permanent beds employing interplanting, decoy crops, biological pest control, and various water-conservation experiments. Perennial flowers and herbs are laced among the fruits and vegetables for added color, but more importantly, for the flavor they will add to the crops and their pest-deterring benefits. The livestock program—a milk cow and four pigs—is based on 12 hectares (30 acres) of pasture. There are plans for another cow, goats, and perhaps a horse.

Farallones not only offers short courses and workshops but is also a college-credited institution. Programs deal with alternative energy and resource recovery, food production, and shelter design and construction. Emphasis may be on either the urban or rural

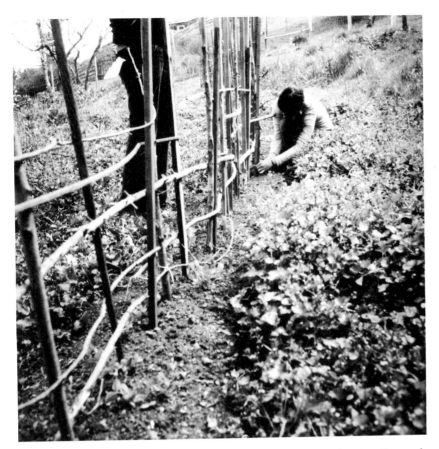

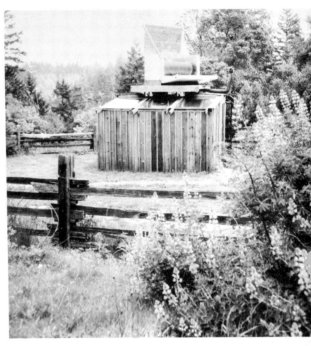

sectors. The educational aim is to help people live better through seeking and implementing new solutions to the integrated problems of energy, economics, and environmental planning.

All aspects of our complex lives are interrelated. At Farallones, these relationships are being focused upon in such a manner as to allow them to complement each other over a period of time. It is fortunate that organizations like the Farallones are showing the way to a restylized life.

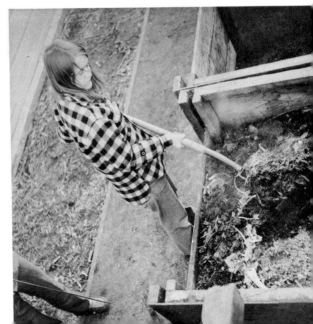

Ecotope

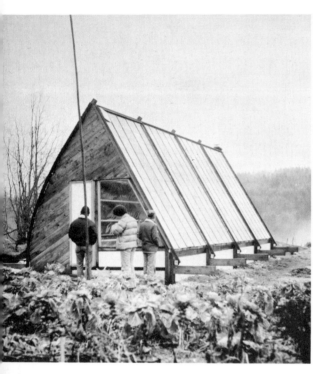

The Ecotope Group is synonymous with energy conservation and alternative activities in and around the Seattle area. Organized in 1971, Ecotope is a nonprofit corporation researching, developing, and demonstrating solar and conservation technologies applicable to the Pacific Northwest. Its activities have ranged from the development of a large methane bioconversion plant at a state institution, to the formulation of a comprehensive energy-conservation plan for the state of Montana. The Group also offers numerous programs and projects for individual adoption.

Tilapia, the vegetarian fish that are a source of experimentation at the New Alchemy Institute (page 98), are also being researched by Ecotope. Jeff Barnes and Howdy Reichmuth designed and constructed a parabolic solar greenhouse at Pragtree, the farm where Ecotope's work is conducted. The arching north wall of the greenhouse scoops sunlight into a Tilapia fish-growing tank located in the north side of the greenhouse. The scooping action of the foil-covered walls increases by two or three times the amount of solar energy penetrating the water. It is really amazing to go from the chill, fog-shrouded fields at 2° C. (35° F.) into a physically comfortable and visually pleasing greenhouse that has no fossil-fuel heating system. The projecting beams will eventually hold insulated reflector panels that will further increase solar reflection into the growing area, and when closed at night, prevent excessive heat loss through the glass.

The height of the structure will aid cooling during the summertime. A stack effect will be created by venting out the top, stimulating air circulation and dissipating heat.

The parabolic solar greenhouse aquaculture complex is a good example of a mini-integrated system. The sun provides direct-gain heating for feeding plants and heating water. The water also provides a certain amount of humidity. The fish respire carbon dioxide, providing a healthy environment for the plants, and the plants, in turn, give off oxygen that the fish can use. The intricacy of nature's webs is incredible, and even more unbelievable is that we can become a vital part of that amazing structure.

A sylvan outhouse, located in an easily accessible yet private area, contains a composting toilet—a clivus multrum. The workings of the clivus are explained under whole-life systems at the Farallones (page 94). An important point is that saner, resource-producing rather than energy-consuming alternatives are available for people far from sewer lines or for those who do not want septic tanks. Composting toilets are nonpolluting, use no water, and can be installed almost anywhere.

The small cabin that serves as temporary living quarters for people working at Pragtree has been fitted with a thermosyphon solar hot-water-heating system. Properly designed, the thermosyphon is an excellent domestic hot-water alternative that has widespread application throughout the United States.

Ecotope consultants have engaged in a variety of educational activities to enable people to help others. Their teachings are having the desired chain-reaction effect. The teacher-teaching project at Canyon Park Junior High School in Bothell, Washington, is one such program. The focal point of Ecotopian education is a passively heated solar greenhouse located out the back door of the science wing at the junior high. This greenhouse uses a combination concrete and water-storage system to provide auxiliary heat over and above the direct-gain heating a greenhouse normally receives. The north wall—18 kilotron (20 tons) and 30 centimeters (12 inches) thick—is a pea-gravel-filled concrete block wall. It is insulated externally and covered with wooded siding. The prediction is that the wall will provide 60 percent of the necessary auxiliary heat. The shelves along the vertical south windows will hold 200 clear polyvinyl water-filled bags, each with the capacity to hold 28.3 cubic centimeters (1 cubic foot) of water. These bags will allow light for nourishing plant growth to pass through while absorbing heat for reradiation after sundown. The remaining 40 percent of the heat will be supplied by the water bags. The south windows will be covered by insulated reflector panels similar to those to be used on the Pragtree greenhouse. This house will extend the six-month growing season to ten months.

As an institution, Ecotope is doing much for the Pacific Northwest. Workshop courses, political involvement, and the visible projects have shown people feasible ways of helping themselves. All Ecotope's activities have been carried out in an economically unselfish manner, with the good of people and the environment as the primary focus.

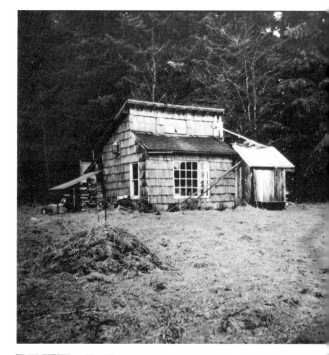

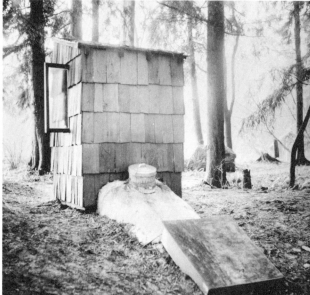

New Alchemy Institute

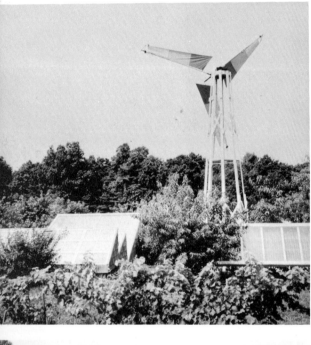

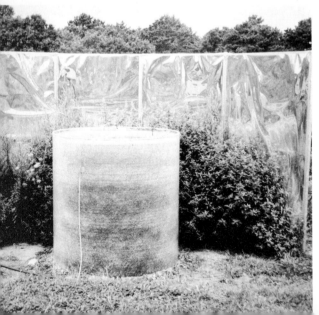

Medieval times witnessed the "miracles" of the alchemist, a cross between a philosopher and a scientist, who reputedly had the power to change something common into something precious, especially base metals into gold. Alchemists do not exist today, but perhaps their place has been taken by a group of people who call themselves the New Alchemists.

The New Alchemy Institute is a nonprofit, loosely-knit organization of men, women, and their children who are performing modern alchemy with the precious forms of energy produced by the sun, wind, water, and land. How do the "Alchies," as they are sometimes called, do this? Simply by exercising a gentle stewardship over natural sources of energy.

In their quest to redirect us from our present ecological insanity, the Alchies have established research centers in various climatic zones of the world. These small independent centers in New England, on the West Coast, and in the tropics allow diverse experimentation in the relationships between the environment and human beings. The New England research station, on Cape Cod, Massachusetts, is a series of integrated models of the approaches being taken to develop strategies of stewardship. These models are built around structural units or "arks." An ark doesn't resemble Noah's, but it does attempt to provide for all of the needs of the organisms that inhabit it.

The miniark, one of the Alchemists' earlier ventures, serves as an excellent example of how a self-contained, integrated system operates. In this miniark highly productive and tasteful Tilapia, or St. Peter's fish, are reared as a food source. Certain needs of the fish are met by capturing wind with a sail-wing windmill that pumps and aerates water. Warming the water through direct solar gain and solar collectors keeps these tropical fish comfortable and encourages them to grow more rapidly. A built-in biological filter in a separate tank removes the fishes' toxic wastes. The wastes then become a resource. They are used to culture algae, which serves as an inhouse food source for the fish.

A separate set of shallow pools is used to culture midge larvae. These nonbiting insects are indigenous to the area and will readily lay their eggs on burlap strips in these manure-fertilized pools. After the eggs hatch, the midge larvae are fed to the Tilapia. The Alchies haven't solved the perpetual-motion problem, but they are producing a crop with only limited ties to the fossil-fuel system under which most of us operate.

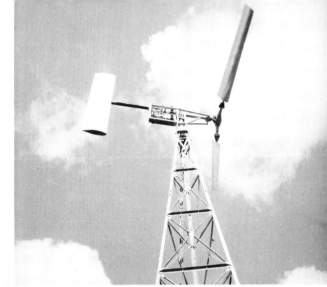

The miniark is extremely subtle, and perhaps that is why it emulates nature so well. For example, a stream is more productive than a pond, and the sail wing provides the "stream lining" for the miniark. It is a polyculture, as opposed to a monoculture. More than one species of fish is stocked to feed at different niches in the system. By carefully selecting organisms, an ecosystem can be designed in which numerous kinds of plants and animals are grown simultaneously without materially reducing one another's growth.

The Alchemists' focus is directed toward small, human-scale projects. If we ever suffer a catastrophe of some kind, the Alchies want people to be able to provide for themselves in a variety of ways. Their research in both conventional and unusual areas is termed *appropriate technology* because it will benefit everyone. They do not necessarily favor complete self-sufficiency, but a bioregional strategy that will enable an area to provide for itself. It is also important to note that the New Alchemists aim to achieve their ends with the least possible environmental destruction.

One of their most creative and simple offerings is the solar algae pond. These fiberglass cylinders may be as large as 3000 liters. That pictured here is about 1700 liters. The ponds are semiclosed fish-growing tanks that can be placed anywhere—though they perform better in the house, where the sun will strike them, because they become heat-storage sinks in addition to fish ponds.

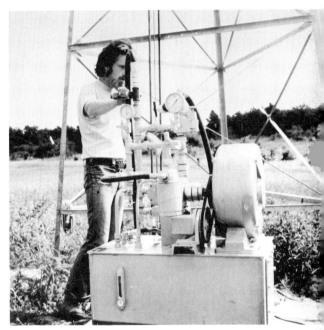

Another project, more oriented to group needs, is the Hydrowind, a wind generator that uses hydraulic principles to produce an electric current. When the wind blows, fluid is sucked up from a reservoir on the ground to a hydraulic pump on the windmill tower. The rotating blades activate the pump, which pressurizes the fluid, which is pumped down to an electric generator on the ground. Perhaps the first of its kind, the Hydrowind has the advantages of a horizontal-axis windmill without a generator on the tower, and also allows direct-drive hookup for doing mechanical work. It is shown here in its second day of operation; its potential power output is estimated at 8–10 kilowatts. This type of generator will be used to produce electricity for the New Alchemists' most ambitious project to date: the Prince Edward Island Ark (PEI). Pictured is the Cape Cod Ark, a smaller version of what is being done on Prince Edward Island.

Maybe the PEI Ark is the ultimate in bioshelters. However, I see it as just an early step and believe the Alchemists will proceed toward even more appropriate alternative technology. The PEI Ark is currently under construction in Charlottetown, Prince Edward Island, Canada. In addition to the wind-power application, the ark will be solar heated, contain aquaculture and agriculture areas, and provide residential space for a family of four. Nancy Todd best describes what the ark will be in *The Journal of the New Alchemists,* No. 3: "It is our intention that the Prince Edward Island ark be productive enough to generate sufficient income to provide its residents with a new economic base. Such structures might conceivably initiate new concepts of household economics, income and self-sufficiency. Another factor underlying the ark concept was that

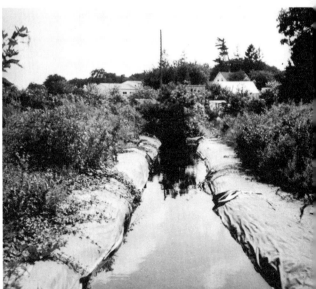

99

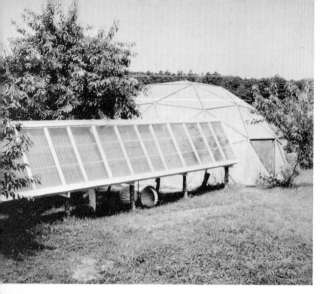

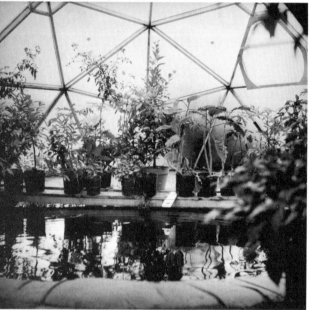

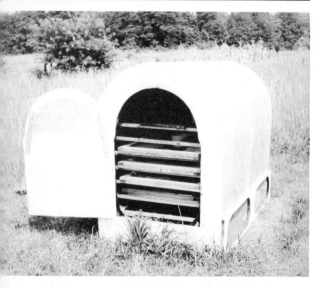

once built, it would not impinge heavily on the external world by polluting neighboring ecosystems, consuming scarce and expensive fuels, or utilizing nuclear power. Rather than stimulate growing energy needs, arks might lead to conserver concepts as yet only dimly foreseen.''

Another area of extensive research is associated with the small-scale farm maintained at Cape Cod. Although the farm is garden-sized, the research is being directed toward agriculture in general. Projects include seeking varieties of vegetables that have genetic resistance to insect pests, and companion plantings (with the vegetables) of herbs and flowers to trap or repel these pests. This lush and productive minifarm was achieved without benefit of commercial fertilizers, insecticides, or herbicides.

The garden and the aquaculture activities have been integrated by using turnover water from the fish ponds for irrigation. Not only are these waters laden with nutrients, but they also contain substances that conserve soil moisture. These moisture-conserving substances bear further research because of their possible use with crops grown in arid areas.

Numerous other hard- and software applications serve as ties between all the minisystems being studied. A solar crop-drier with a dehumidifier aids in the preservation of the crops. Extensive composting and a waste recycling system complement Mother Nature's return cycles. A savonius rotor is used to pump water for garden irrigation. Bug lights attract and kill nighttime insects, which are, in turn, fed to the fish. The mind-boggling array of examples and ideas emanating from this nonhierarchical group of people, whose projects are supported by contributions and their own hard work, is endless.

The point is that the work of the Alchemists is holistic. All the various facets of their research are woven together to become part of a total yet diverse system. Visual examples at New Alchemy, the teaching activities of the New Alchemists, and their publications have catalyzed people throughout the world. The Alchemists' explorations will form the core of a bio-regional variability that can be our alternative future—one that is humble, restorative, and ecologically wise.

Of Straw and Rocks

Sanford Beck is a farmer in northern California who employs both modern technological developments and time-tested methods to make his farming operation less energy consumptive.

He places 5-ton straw bales, from harvested grain that was once burned as waste, on the open range to supply a constant wintertime feed supply for the cattle. Not only is this a source of inexpensive feed, but it also eliminates the unpleasant winter chore of feeding range cattle. An additional benefit to the cattle are the cantilevered shelters from the elements that are formed as the cattle eat into these bales.

If a tree is planted very near the large granite boulders that are plentiful on the farm, it will have its own natural heat-storage sink. The rock, heated by the constant sun, reradiates that heat to the atmosphere at night, often preventing the temperature from dropping to a level damaging to trees. It almost seems Mother Nature is offering a trade—solar hot rocks for smudge-pot fuel oil.

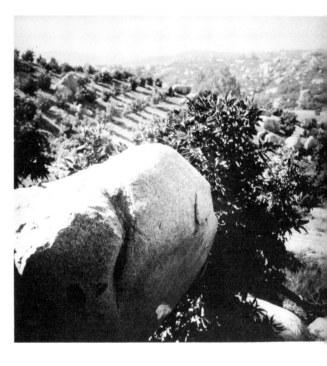

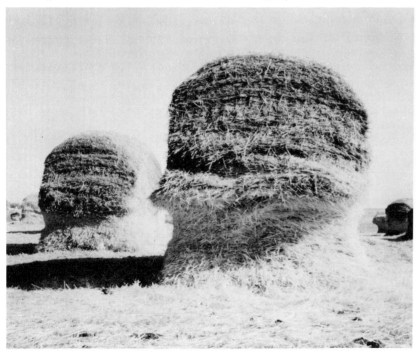

Hager's Solar Abode

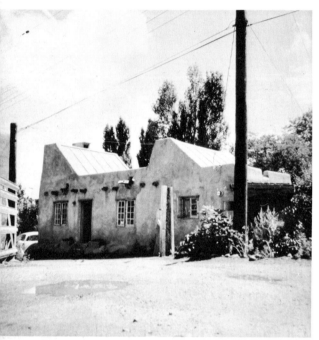

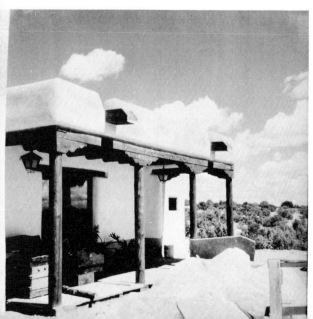

Santa Fe is a beautiful old city with architecture in the traditions of the early Spaniards and American Indians. Some of the oldest buildings in the United States can be found in this venerable city, which has attracted artisans, entrepreneurs, environmentalists, and people who simply want to enjoy the big clear skies of New Mexico. But Santa Fe is growing, and urban growth, unless it is well planned, can become a cancer destroying the very tissue of a city.

It is refreshing to find a builder/developer who is committed to constructing energy-conserving homes. Richard Hager has built a made-to-order passive solar home for a young family that he hopes will provide the impetus for a new subdivision, perhaps to be called an "energy park."

The Hager-built home is unfinished. A solar greenhouse will be added to the south side of the house. The greenhouse will provide food and heat to the primary living area. An adobe fireplace built on this wall will heat both the house and the greenhouse when there is insufficient sun. Another interesting addition is a glassed-in sitting room attached to the southwest portion of the house. This room will pass on its late afternoon heat to the master bedroom. The very mass of the adobe walls and the proper distribution of windows add to the energy-conserving ability of the house.

Small nuclei of architects and builders will eventually prove the inevitability of home construction based initially and primarily on energy-conservation principles.

Solar Pioneers:
Florence and Peter van Dresser

Like our forefathers, Florence and Peter van Dresser migrated west, only their move—from New York to New Mexico—was made in 1949. Before coming to New Mexico, Peter had been deeply involved in the prewar Decentralist movement and wrote extensively on a variety of related subjects, including the small-scale biotechnic theory, which advocates the redistribution of population into smaller, more humane, and more efficient communities. In an article published in a 1938 issue of *Free America,* he predicted the coming energy crisis and discussed most of the alternatives now being explored.

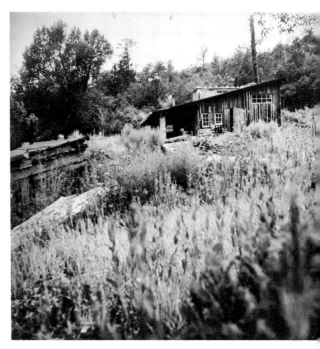

He dropped out of architectural school in 1930 because he felt that what was being taught was not relevant to the urgent problems of the near future. (He doesn't think the situation has changed much in the last forty-seven years.) He lived for several years aboard his ketch, and then during his first homesteading venture on the borders of the Everglades in southern Florida he fabricated and erected solar water heaters.

When he and Florence migrated to New Mexico, their philosophy began to solidify. In north-central New Mexico the van Dressers have evolved a life-style that has enabled them to integrate their lives with the environment. Their adopted home is the quiet community of El Rito. Here they have tried to work constructively with the local people and with government agencies, but, more importantly, they have set an example of how people can become self-reliant within the constraints placed on them by the community and the environment. A small village restaurant (which was recently sold), an energy-conserving house, and a small cooperative farm outside El Rito have all demonstrated the message Peter delivers in his book, *A Landscape for Humans.*

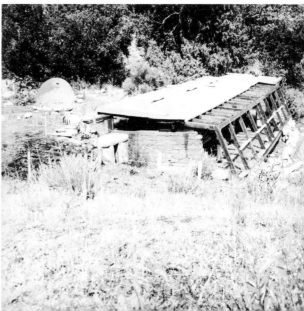

To the van Dressers, solar application is but one approach to redesigning our lives on a more human scale. They feel that we must also develop local and regional autonomy so we can create communities with logistical patterns that enable people to live well while using much less energy. Social changes must occur, but in an evolutionary, nontraumatic way. If this type of transformation is to be realized, it must begin at the periphery and then blend into the mainstream of society.

According to most records, the van Dressers own the second-oldest continuously-heated solar house in the United States (George Lof of Denver has the oldest). In 1958 Peter retrofitted an adobe

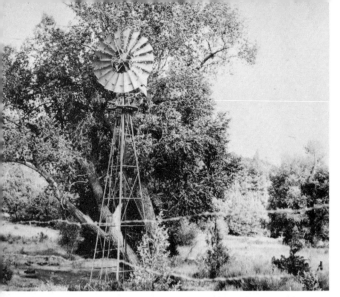

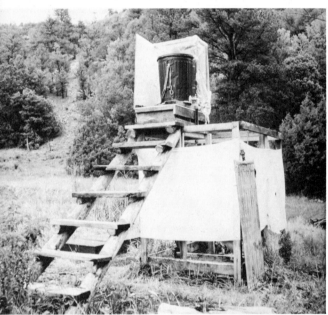

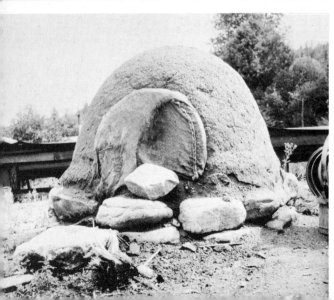

building in the old section of Santa Fe into a respectable solar home. The building's long axis ran north and south—the wrong way for the most efficient sun gathering. It is rather difficult to reorient a building, so Peter adapted the building to the situation. Two air-type collector panels, totaling 21 square meters (230 square feet), were installed on the south-facing roof sections at 45-degree angles. Actually, solar panels can be inclined on an existing flat adobe roof simply by cementing more brick at the desired angle. The collectors are glazed with a single layer of glass that rests 2.5 centimeters (1 inch) above a black painted sheet of heat-absorbing steel. The two sets of collectors each heat a different part of the 58-square-meter (630-square-foot) single-story dwelling. The larger collector to the north serves the living area by two 13-centimeter (5-inch) ducts that run from the collector to a sand pit under the brick floor. Through this 30-centimeter (12-inch) thick layer of sand, 7.5-centimeter (3-inch) horizontal pipes on 40-centimeter (16-inch) centers have been laid. These pipes infuse their heat into the sand, from which the heat is reradiated back into the house. The 80-watt blowers direct the air from the collectors to the pipes in the sand. The south end of the pipes discharges warm air directly into the room.

The smaller collector to the south works the same way to heat the kitchen and bathroom. The hot air is blown into a pit of stones 2 centimeters (3.12 inches) in diameter. The stone pit is insulated with pumice blocks. An air-to-water heat exchanger in this duct also heats water for domestic use. The blowers run only when the differential thermostat notes about a 7° C. (12° F.) difference between the collector and the storage temperatures. In seventeen years of operation about 65 percent of all heating has been solar.

At present, Peter is drawing on his years of experience with solar energy to construct a larger house for himself and his wife in El Rito. This house is described in *Homegrown Sundwellings*, a book in which Peter sums up the results of two years of research and experimentation by the Sundwellings team, of which he was director-coordinator. The team was established to systematize the successful techniques for indigenous solar construction evolved in New Mexico and similar semiarid regions.

The Potrero de Abajo is a 20-hectare (50-acre) valley owned by the van Dressers and located 6.5 kilometers (3.5 miles) north of El Rito. Many of their early years in New Mexico were spent here. The Potrero has attracted a gathering of people seeking a community-scale, self-reliant life. Peter has long felt that the present generation of ecology-motivated counter-culturalists tends to overemphasize gadgetry (in which category he includes dome habitats, most wind and methane generators, a variety of solar-powered widgets, and the like). He hopes in Potrero the emphasis will be on the gradual development of the valley as an organic, ecologically managed productive whole characterized by careful management of land, water, and vegetation, microclimate modification, and efficient living quarters.

Individual reasons for advocating people-scale technology vary from a savior self-image to just plain self-fulfillment. Throughout this country there is a new zeal for finding a way of life more in harmony with nature.

Briefly, the Potrero (still in the embryonic stage, considering its long-term objectives) has extensive garden plots that are refurbished by compost, animal manure, and crop rotation. The community also has a solar crop-dryer to preserve the produce for later consumption. A large greenhouse of adobe and local wood has extended the growing season and may help in heating the house. A windmill pumps the valley's irrigation, drinking, and bathing water. An outdoor solar shower, suitable for this particular situation, is used in the summertime, and a solar-warmed composting toilet is near completion. In the future wind-electric or other appropriate units of technology will no doubt contribute to the advancement of this community.

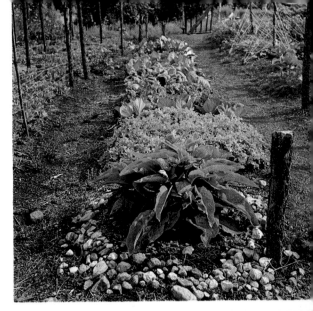

The Potrero de Abajo community is really attempting to reestablish a relationship with nature we had thought lost forever. The old villages of the Southwest were constructed around the *acequia madre*—the mother ditch. Water was the lifeblood of the village, and the ditch was the artery of conveyance. Given the technology of the day, no one could move far from the *acequia madre,* so each community was a close-knit group of people working to make the locality supply all their needs.

Super technology has all but destroyed the small community, and we are reaching the point of diminishing returns in mass living. Peter van Dresser has studied the modern laws and institutions that are expediting the destruction of traditional communities rather than helping them innovate for the future. In *A Landscape for Humans* he concludes with a resolution he presented to the 1970 International Design Conference in Aspen, Colorado, which was unanimously adopted. A part of that resolution reads:

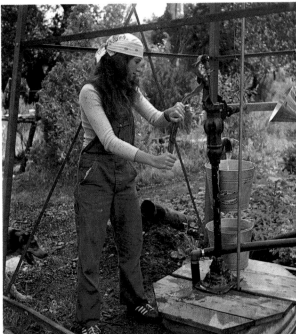

> *A substantial portion of our social effort must be directed toward the revitalization of the entire range of smaller rural and provincial communities. . . . Research on technology appropriate to communities of this type such as construction with abundant and cost-free indigenous materials; intensive agriculture, food production and storage; utilization of solar, wind, and other nonpolluting and nonconsumptive energy sources; close recycling of waste products for maintenance of organic fertility; miscellaneous essential small-scale industries using local resources [must be done].*

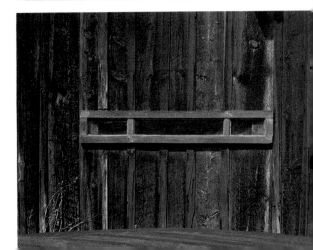

Earthmind

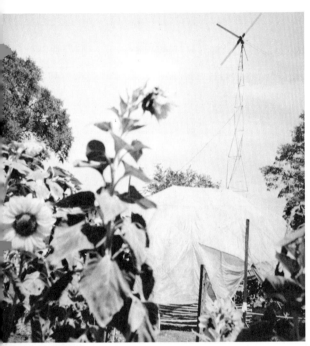

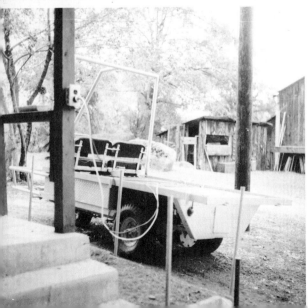

Earthmind is the idea for an alternative community taking shape. This nonprofit group is at present composed of three people—Mark Dankoff, Michael Hackleman, and Vanessa Naumann—who, as researchers, writers, and educators, want to share their findings and thoughts with others as concerned as they are with alternative energy.

A visit to the Earthmind temporary headquarters in the Sierra foothills near the gateway to Yosemite Valley, California, is an immediate visual experience. Perched atop what resembles a crooked tower is a 1500-watt Wincharger electric wind generator. The octahedron-module tower is based on the geodesic dome principle, and like the dome, derives its strength from the eight triangles that make up each octahedron module. The 14.3-meter (47-foot) tower gives the optical illusion of undulating its way skyward, when, in fact, it is straight. It is made from 2.5-centimeter (1-inch) electrical metallic tubing (EMT). Tubing size varies according to the height of the tower and the weight of the generator it is to support. O-M towers have numerous advantages, including strength, light weight, simplicity, and ease of construction, and they are less expensive to construct than conventional three- or four-leg towers.

The wind generator is wired into a bank of storage batteries in the back porch of the house. These provide the 32-volt current needed to operate various kinds of equipment and appliances. What kind of appliances? "Ever eat a wind-powered waffle?" Michael asked. Electricity from the same battery bank charges a retrofitted electric vehicle. While it is an excellent workhorse for activities on the 16-hectare (40-acre) farm, the little unit is hardly a legitimate street vehicle, so the people at Earthmind are considering building their own electric car.

One characteristic of concerned communities such as Earthmind is their holistic approach to meeting basic needs. In conjunction with their energy work, agriculture and gardening activities are important focal points. The parachute-covered conduit dome provides another link in the chain of self-reliance. The "orangehouse," if properly ventilated, is a good place to start winter vegetables.

The Earthmind people strongly believe in proper diet and nutrition. A pedal-powered flour mill enables them to grind their own wheat in an energy-conserving manner. Mark has taken a bicycle

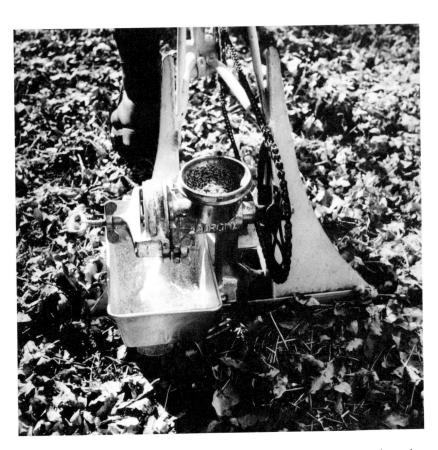

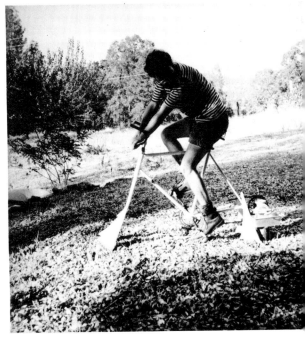

and converted it into a grinder that works much faster and easier than the old hand-cranked mills.

Although Earthmind has been at its present location only since May 1976, the group has already become part of the community. People often get the idea that alternative communities are seeking a hermetic self-sufficiency. In most cases that could not be farther from the truth: the energy exchanges between friends and neighbors are vital to reeducating and *spreading the word.*

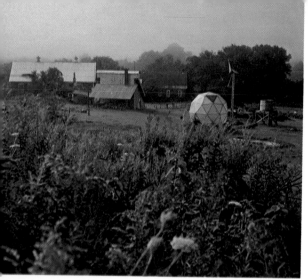

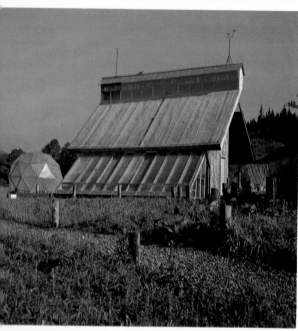

The Social Ecology Experience: Goddard College

Much of the work being done to promote and teach practical solutions to environmental and energy-related problems is taking place at our learning institutions. Rather conventional research programs are being carried out by large state universities, but some of the more important and interesting approaches are being taken at small private schools like Goddard College.

Goddard's Institute for Social Ecology in Plainfield, Vermont, was founded in 1974 by Murray Bookchin in collaboration with Dan Chodorkoff. Theoretical and practical approaches are taken in introducing students to various subjects, including ecology, agriculture, wind power, solar applications, aquaculture, and waste treatment. During the summer between 100 and 150 students are treated to the inspiring discussions provided by guest instructors like John and Nancy Todd, Karl Hess, Steve Baer, Eugene Eccli, Robert Reines, Richard Merrill, Hans Meyer, and Wilson Clark, who are invited to lecture on their work and experience.

Goddard conducts its programs on Cate Farm, an old farmstead that is being retrofitted into an ecological self-sufficient unit. The farm's setting, with the Winooski River meandering by on the east and hills jutting up on the west, provides a beautiful backdrop for the wind towers, domes, and solar buildings that have been erected. The staff at Goddard—Bookchin, Chodorkoff, Charles Woodard, Scott Nielsen, Richard Gottlieb, Steven Capron, among others—is responsible for seeing the Institute's projects to completion. What is being accomplished on campus is a tribute to those involved, because Goddard, unlike other institutions, is not blessed with a huge research budget.

The Goddard projects are a series of life-support systems. The building with the steeply inclined south-facing wall is dubbed the Solar-Heated Wind-Powered Aquaculture Complex (SHWPAC). The southern wall contains 37 square meters (396 square feet) of Kalwall-glazed trickle-type solar collector panels. Gottlieb noted that the structurally simple collectors heated 4500 kilograms (10,000 pounds) of water 2° F. in thirty minutes—which is about 17,640 calories (70,000 BTUs) per hour, or about half the heat necessary to accommodate a typical, poorly insulated 93-square-meter (1000-square-foot) home. (This rapid heat gain was a morning reading

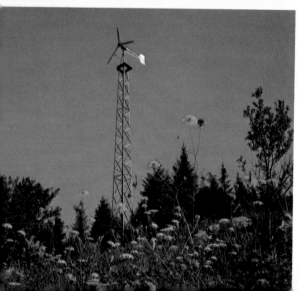

taken prior to water-temperature stabilization.) A 5240-liter (1310-gallon) concrete hot-water storage tank is located inside the SHWPAC, as well as a wood stove for both space heating and backup for the hot-water tank. The 1800-watt Jacobs wind generator provides electricity for lighting the structure. Since the generator produces 32-volt electricity, an inverter will have to be installed before the 110-volt pumps can be operated by the Jacobs. At present, crayfish are being cultured in the aquaculture part of the complex. Their water is heated by a heat-exchange system through the heat-storage tank. Eventually plants will also be grown, and there is space for additional experimental equipment and classes on an upper level.

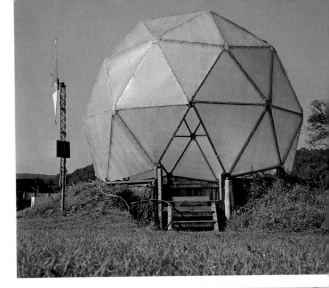

As a result of recent internal structural changes and added insulation, the Institute staff believes that the structure will prove remarkably efficient in cold climates. According to their calculations, an interior temperature of 19° C. (65° F.) can be maintained when exterior temperatures fall as low as −9° C. (15° F.), and days are only 40 percent sunny.

The Kalwalled dome adds a touch of futurama to the landscape. It contains a circular plywood fish tank that houses fish species indigenous to the area. (According to Bookchin, "we hope to design our operations in such a way that we can develop a breeding stock.") A pump circulates the water through this simulated riverine arrangement. There's a feeling among Goddard's aquaculturists that using indigenous aquatic organisms is a more practical approach to producing proteins than importing exotic specimens.

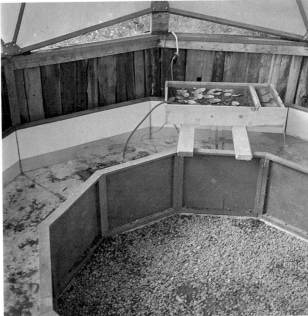

A prairie windmill is expected to be the primary source for pumping irrigation water under drought conditions. Irrigation of the experimental agricultural plots and large organic garden is frequently unnecessary. These farming endeavors are under the capable direction of Charles Woodard, and the cropping philosophy is based on producing high yields of quality foods using natural systems of nutrient supply. Similar-sized plots of the same soil type are planted with the same crops. One is fertilized with commercially available chemical fertilizer; the second, with organic compost; and the last, with slurry, a liquefied manure. Yields are measured, and a chemical analysis of the crops compares protein content, enzyme activity, and vitamin levels.

Gary Kah, a staff member in 1976, has done much to prove that organic wastes are essential resources. With his guidance, students at Goddard have designed and constructed a composting toilet (which has been installed in the Cate Farm house) and a methane generator. The semiexperimental methane generator, which has a Plexiglas viewport on top, is continuous-flowing and is made almost entirely of recycled materials. A capacity of 900 liters (225 gallons) will produce about 1130 liters (40 cubic feet) of bio-gas per day. (It takes about 226 liters (8 cubic feet) of bio-gas to cook a simple meal.) Eventually the bio-gas will be used to heat water in a gas hot-water heater.

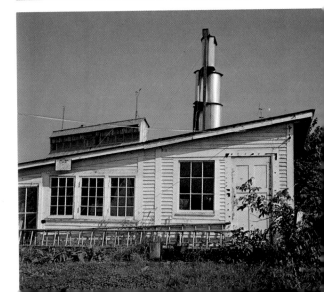

The Savonius rotor is an S-shaped wind-speed device. Since the vertical wind machines have low rpm's, they are most often used to convert wind energy into mechanical energy. The Savonius mounted on the shed next to the farmhouse will probably be used to stir the

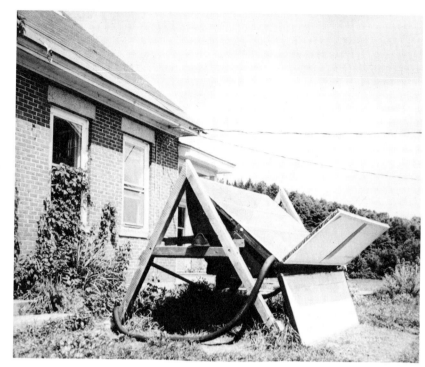

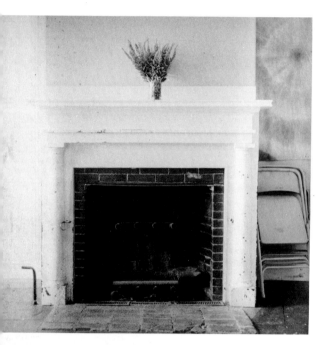

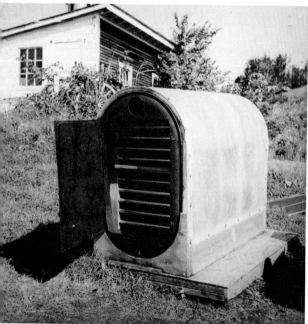

manure slurry in the methane digestor.

The Institute's other projects are too numerous to be discussed here, but several should at least be mentioned. A rebuilt FES Delta (trademark) concentrating solar collector is used for heating water in the farmhouse. A thermograte was built to increase the efficiency of the fireplace, which was retrofitted with a venting system to further increase efficiency. A south brick wall was painted black, vented on top and bottom, and glassed. A device like this serves as a simple passive heat collector, and is actually a mini-Trombe wall.

What is actually happening at the Social Ecology Institute's Cate Farm installation is an evolving integrated system. When all the ingredients have been added, Cate Farm will be an example of an almost self-sufficient farm and homestead.

The Organic Gardening Experimental Farm

Maxatawny, an Indian word whose translation is "Creek Where the Bears Walk," is the site of Rodale Press's new Organic Gardening Experimental Farm (OGEF). This land was originally farmed in 1819 by a German family. Rodale purchased the chemically farmed acreage in 1972. The acquisition of these 122 hectares (305 acres) in eastern Pennsylvania has opened the door to more extensive research in agriculture production based on simpler and saner techniques. The farm fits nicely into other Rodale activities. It is on the not particularly fertile soils of this farm in Emmaus that Rodale's Research and Development people have set up their Home Utilities Workshop to test small-scale gardening and farming tools and equipment. Devices like seed and bean sprouters and food driers are tested in the Fitness House Kitchen, also in Emmaus, which uses food produced on the farm. Rodale's findings are published and disseminated throughout the world.

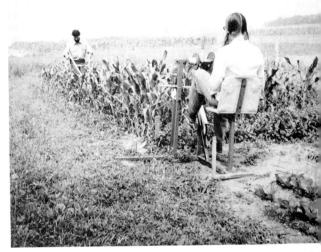

The device that is cultivating one of the farm's experimental plots is Research and Development's (R&D's) Energy Cycle. At Rodale there is a feeling that the small-scale family farm is coming back. Research by Rural America, Inc., indicates that a new breed of younger farmers with smaller acreages is successfully adopting energy-saving methods. The Cycle is one example of an appropriately-sized piece of equipment that will help these farmers become economically competitive by freeing them from their dependence on expensive motors and fossil-fuel energy. The 74.5 watts (0.1 horsepower) that our legs are capable of generating can grind, juice, crop food, pump water, churn butter, turn a lathe, and even generate electricity. The Cycle was still being debugged when I was at Rodale, but by the time you read this it will probably be available for sale.

A $300 per-season heating bill for a 23.8-square-meter (256-square-foot) greenhouse prompted the Rodale people to build a solar greenhouse. Unlike the other solar greenhouses discussed throughout this book, Rodale's performance has been monitored. Although greenhouses are traditionally constructed of transparent material, they never receive direct sunlight from the north side. Since it is a simple matter to compensate for the diffuse light available through the north wall, it seems logical to insulate this portion of the house to reduce heat loss. At OGEF a portion of the roof and the east and west walls, as well as the north wall, are insulated with 19 centimeters (7.5 inches) of cellulose fiber. The plants are vig-

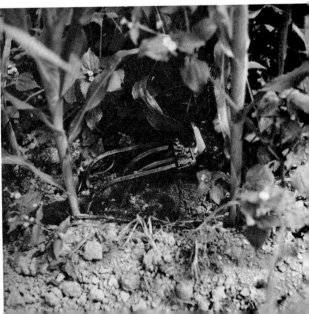

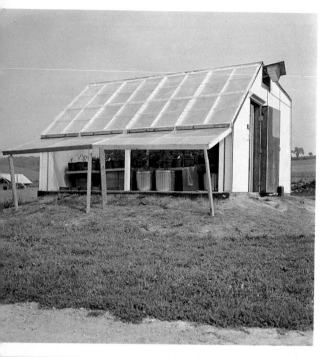

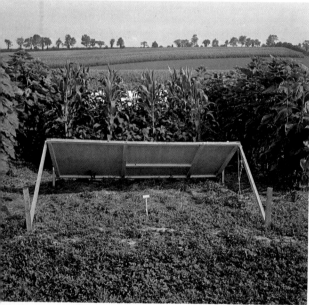

orous, straight, and tall. In the winter the sun rises and sets so far south on the horizon that clear side walls would give little extra light. The most effective sunlight for heating occurs between 9:00 A.M. and 3:00 P.M. in midwinter, and that shines through the clear south wall. To prevent heat loss through the ground, 5 centimeters (2 inches) of plastic foam sheets have been placed under 60 centimeters (2 feet) of an earth floor. The heat-storage system consists of a bank of metal containers painted black, filled with water, and stacked against the interior north wall. This thermal sink stores heat for use when the sun isn't shining and also helps to cool the greenhouse when it overheats. A small fan in the peak of the ceiling can be used to force hot air over the water-storage area and reduce air temperature considerably. On a sunny day a greenhouse such as this will gather 44 kilowatt-hours (150,000 BTUs) of energy. Very little of this energy is necessary to keep the house warm, so it seems logical to capture and store it for later use.

Other solar work being researched includes the testing of four solar panels. The performances of these panels are being metered in the R & D lab, and from these tests a panel for more widespread use on the farm and in farmhouses will be selected. Solar reflector fences are being used in crop plots to stretch the growing seasons and keep the soil a little warmer. In an interplanting trial—which will be discussed in more detail—soybean yields were reduced when planted with corn because they were overshadowed by the corn. Solar fences will be used to reflect light into the lower soybeans. Rodale has found that if soybeans receive sufficient light during the flowering stage, their yields will not be affected.

The batch methane digestor is solar heated to speed gas production by the bacteria. A portable insulated reflector panel on the front of the unit increases daytime radiation and is closed at night to retain heat. As bio-gas is generated, it is piped and stored in a water-submerged tank. At its peak, the digestor was producing enough gas to operate one Bunsen burner for eight hours a day, with an average output of 0.34 cubic meters (12 cubic feet) per day. The methane is used in a Bunsen burner to distill water for use in the R & D laboratory.

A "hot box" is based on the thermos concept. A hot, but not cooked, stew or soup is placed in this foil-lined, heavily insulated box. The residual heat from the dish is trapped, and it cooks itself. Temperatures of 74° C. (165° F.) for four hours have been recorded, which is sufficient to cook the food.

The longtime research by Rodale on agriculture alternatives is impressive, but their current work is even more extensive. Interplanting—the planting together of crops that complement each other—may have far-reaching effects on yields and natural fertility systems. Planting corn, a high nitrogen feeder, with soybeans, a crop capable of fixing atmospheric nitrogen in the soil, is an example of one such system. The denser leaf canopy created by interplanting shades out weeds, conserves moisture by reducing evaporation, and captures more solar energy. Other plant pairings now under experimentation are carrots with sugar peas, cabbage with bush beans, and tomatoes with soybeans.

Nitrogen is a nutrient that plants require in great amounts. Commercial nitrogen fertilizer is an energy-intensive product, and it accounts for about 32 percent of the energy budget for Midwestern corn. At Rodale, efforts are being directed toward using natural, less energy-intensive sources of nitrogen. Legume plants like soybeans, alfalfa, and clovers are well known for their ability to fix atmospheric nitrogen in the soil. But what about such strange-sounding plants as azolla and anabaena? Azolla is a water fern and anabaena is a blue-green algae. Both are found in the rice paddies of Vietnam. Their association seems to be synergistic—that is, when they are planted together, nitrogen fixation is greatly enhanced, thus benefiting the associated rice crop. Rodale hopes to grow these plants in the greenhouse and use them for fertilizer.

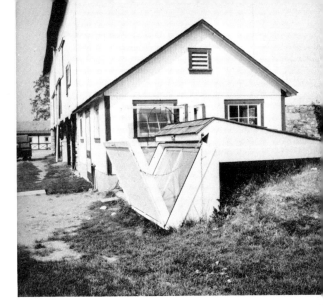

Pleurotus Sajor-Caju sounds like the name of the first Martian on earth. Actually this plant is an edible nitrogen-fixing fungus. The mushroom can be grown on a straw and corncob substrate. After it is harvested and eaten, the substrate is nitrogen rich and can be used as a fertilizer. Still another plant, Koa Haole, a giant Hawaiian perennial legume, can be harvested and used as a nitrogen-rich green manure plant. The leaves and young pods are edible and have a high protein content. These plants are but a few examples of nature's system of plant nutrition and soil fertility that seemed sufficient prior to chemical manipulation of the soil by humans.

Rodale Press has grown into a very large family. In spite of its size, the group has been able to nurture a strong feeling for the land along with a spirit of self-reliance and self-sufficiency. A wide range of new concepts for home and small-farm food production are being explored. Using organic techniques, new crop and livestock species and production technologies are being developed for the gardener and small farmer. As with most of the people investigating alternatives for living, energy conservation and the use of renewable resources are primary objectives of this group.

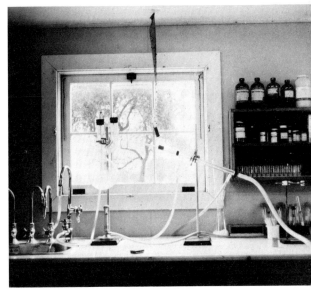

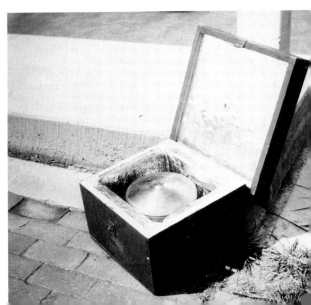

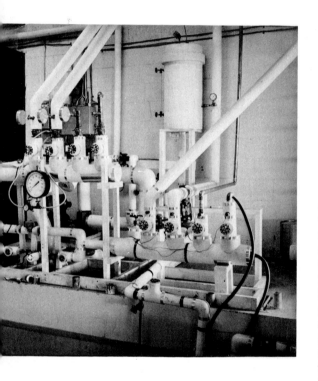

Dairy farming in the United States has changed considerably from the days when cows were hand-milked and milk was stored in 40-liter (10-gallon) cans. Today the business is a highly mechanized bulk enterprise. In spite of mechanization, however, the average dairy in the United States supports only seventy-three cows. Most modern dairy farmers spend considerable amounts of money on energy to heat water, refrigerate milk, and heat their milking facilities in the winter. Dr. Paul Thompson of the USDA and his colleagues felt that solar applications for dairies had enough merit to bear testing, and decided that the tests would be directed toward helping the small dairy farmer.

The USDA dairy at Beltsville, Maryland, is a prototype unit. Its solar system was constructed with materials readily available to farmers. Because it is a test unit, it has more hardware than one might find on a dairy in the future. Four sets of water-type flat-plate collectors are being tested: a single-glazed glass, open-channel trickle type, with a nonselective absorbing surface on the aluminum absorber plate; a single-glazed matte-finish glass with a selective absorber surface on the copper tube, copper-sheet absorber plate; a double-glazed tempered glass with a nonselective absorber coating on the roll-bond aluminum plate; and a double-glazed lexan with a selective coating absorbing surface and an aluminum roll-bond absorber plate. The simultaneous evaluation of four different panels could provide valuable information about the performances of the various types of collectors. The trickle-type collector covers 23.4 square meters (256 square feet), while the other three occupy 20.1 square meters (217 square feet). At the time we photographed the dairy, only two of the four sets of panels had been installed.

The heart of this system is a 37,850-liter (10,000-gallon) underground concrete hot-water storage tank insulated with urethane. A urethane disc floats on the water inside the tank for further insulation. The tank is covered with a fiberglass silo dome. Water from the bottom of the tank is pumped and distributed to each bank of collectors. The warmest water from the top of the tank is pumped into the barn. In the pit of the parlor barn are the conventional hot-water fan-coil space heaters supplied with this solarized water. The heaters are equipped with a thermostat that the milker can control. Hot water to wash and prime cows prior to milking and for cleanup purposes is produced in the following manner: Well water

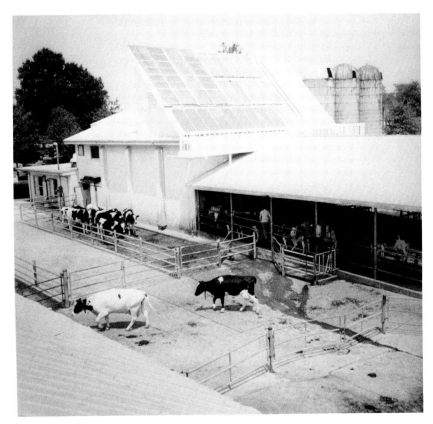

is pumped to a heat exchanger that, in turn, heats the water in a 450-liter (120-gallon) hot-water storage tank. This preheated water then goes into a normal electric hot-water heater for final heating, if necessary. It's a rather straightforward system, so most dairy farmers should be able to install and maintain it themselves.

Dr. Thompson estimates that the solar application (including some equipment for recovery of the waste heat of the refrigeration system) will meet about 75 percent of the average dairy's hot-water needs. The one question dairymen raise is whether solar energy will be economically practicable. Although final results will not be published for about three years, Dr. Thompson has calculated that a capital investment of $3000 could be paid off in six years if the costs of electricity were 4.8 cents per kilowatt-hour or higher. At the end of the six years the farmer would have hot water for the minimal cost of pump operation, and the system should last many more years.

There are other alternatives, and once again they are passive means of conservation. Energy can be conserved by adding insulation to buildings, putting in a water heater that uses waste from the refrigeration tank, and using well water to precool milk. It's up to each dairyman to assess which application would give him the best returns. As fossil fuels become less available and more expensive, dairymen will no doubt become more conscious of energy conservation.

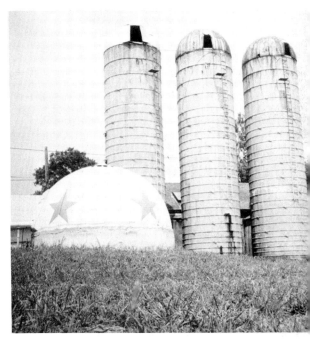

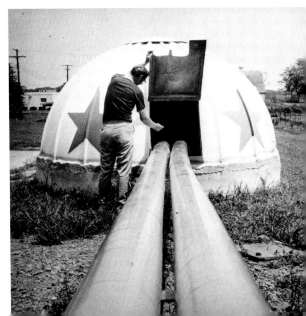

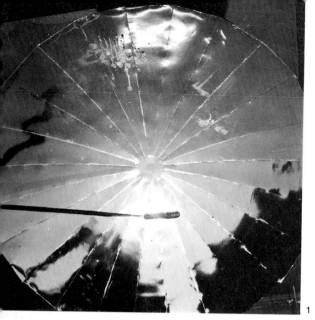

A **parabolic collector** may be used to run a refrigerator, cook hot dogs, or boil water. Constructed by Bill Grim, a San Jose Junior High School teacher who has interested his students in solar energy alternatives, the parabola is aluminized Mylar glued onto a cardboard frame. It served as an example for Bill's students and encouraged them to do some projects on their own. The results— a solar hot dog cooker, an oven, and a solar crock-pot. (1)

Here is a sun-energized device just right for a family outing or weekend trip. This **portable solar cooker** (made of cast aluminum) can be backpacked to any destination and assembled in two minutes. If the sun is even thinking about shining, it will only be a short time before the water is boiling and ready for that mid-morning tea break. There's only one drawback: a $150 price tag. (2)

The compact, collapsible **solar oven** has a wide range of uses: imagine hot apple pie for that midmorning ski break, or warm honey-filled biscuits at a secluded island picnic. The only prerequisite: a few hours of sunlight. (3)

The **crop-dryer** is an example of one of the many designs that a person can build in his or her garage. This dryer takes advantage of the chimney or stack effect. Air heated in the collector, a black-painted quarter-inch plywood sheet glazed with Kalwall, convects into the fruit drying box. As the air cools, it is displaced backward and upward out of the box and into the atmosphere via the chimney. The constant air movement removes moisture from the fruit or vegetable without the use of any additives or direct exposure to sunlight. The dried products retain their natural colors, and vitamin A is not bleached out as it is in sun drying. Collectors of this nature are best suited to dry climates.

Under more humid conditions, some sort of dehumidifier, such as a slanted piece of glass, must be installed to collect the moisture and direct it away. Whatever your climatic situation, this outdoor appliance is a truly useful and simple device. (4)

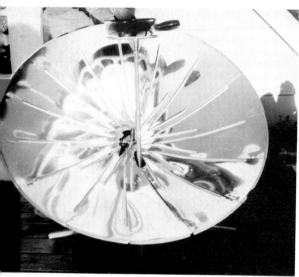

Among certain groups in this country, collective bathing is an everyday experience. The tub pictured here is reputedly the first **solar-heated tub** in Santa Barbara. The 3200 liters (800 gallons) of water contained in this redwood tub are heated by a series of Solarator collector panels mounted on the carport. The tub was solarized because there was no natural gas available, and electrical heating would have been too expensive. Four panels and a 62-watt ($\frac{1}{12}$-horsepower) pump were connected to the existing plumbing system. The result: a steamy success (and the solar equipment has long since paid for itself through energy savings). (5)

Cooking with gas—methane, that is—is one alternative whose application may not be as futuristic as it seems. The production of bio-gas, composed mostly of methane, is a natural biological process that occurs when bacteria attacks organic materials in the absence of oxygen. Given the right conditions, just about anything

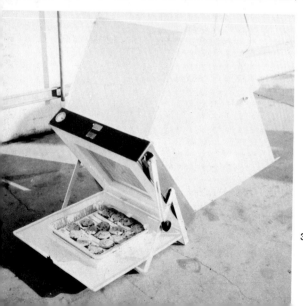

that was once living will produce some methane gas, but certain products seem to work best: the manure from one dairy cow, for instance, will eventually produce 120 cubic feet of gas per day. It takes about 8 cubic feet of methane gas to cook a simple meal.

Methane generation on a small scale is generally impractical. Most of it will take place where there is much organic waste. City waste-treatment plants (there is one in Modesto, California, a town of 85,000 people) are sites of surplus energy production. Many sewage-treatment plants are using their methane for heating and lighting the facility. Cleaning or scrubbing the gas can make it usable in internal combustion engines. Producing internal combustion quality gas is not entirely practical today; in the future, however, this may become a feasible energy alternative. Although most of Modesto's gas is burned off, there is a potential to produce the equivalent of 700 gallons of gasoline per week. In 1970 the United States produced from urban waste 1.36 trillion ft^3 of 1000 BTU/ft^3 methane gas. This is 40 million liters (10 million gallons) worth of gasoline annually, and does not include manure and most other agricultural wastes.

Mother Nature left all this energy in organic materials so that they would eventually dissipate (that's part of her recycling process). Perhaps human intervention in this natural process would not harm nature and would be advantageous to people. It's only a matter of time before the agricultural- and waste-treatment sectors, areas that produce energy resources, will be forced into becoming more energy self-reliant. Methane gas production offers one practical means of attaining that end. (6)

San Diego Gas and Electric . . . and Solar? Can alternative energy remain a cottage industry? Large companies like Lockheed and Grumman, and public utilities like San Diego Gas and Electric (SDG&E), believe they must become vitally involved before alternatives will become economically available in large quantities. It is inevitable that corporate enterprise will play an increasing role in the distribution of these goods and services, and it is hoped that big business will see the desirability of meeting regional and climatic needs because alternative energy applications work best when they are conceived with a true feeling for the area. To achieve a long-range economical net energy balance, corporations must also seek the cooperation of the "backyard inventor" and the alternative energy cottage industry.

If solar energy is to be economically competitive in southern California, all performance parameters must be collected and analyzed. Because a system works well for an individual does not necessarily mean that a public utilities company will find it an economically wise investment. San Diego Gas and Electric is evaluating the performance of solar energy at several private homes in the San Diego area. Atop the company office buildings in downtown San Diego is an extensive solar-panel test yard. Chuck Lischer, who is in charge of the yard, is discovering which panels really perform. Inventors are sending their collector devices to the company to be evaluated. All experimentation is being conducted according to the National Bureau of Standards solar guidelines, which insures greater validity and consistency in the data. The

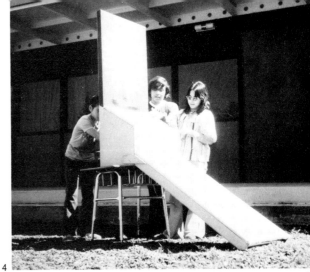

4

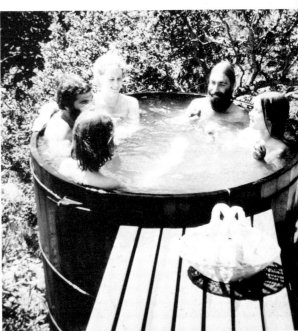

5

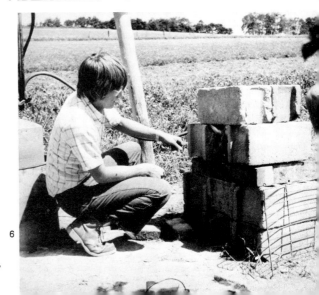

6

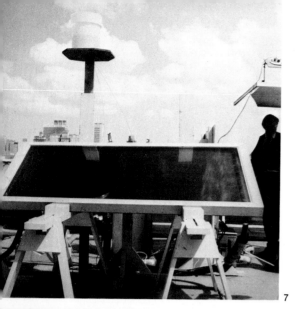

7

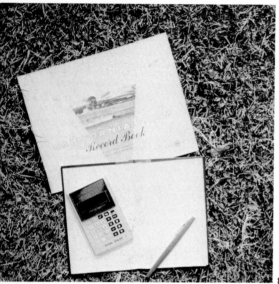

8

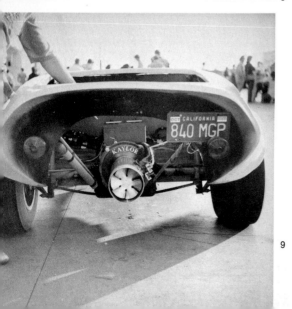

9

pioneer work that San Diego Gas is doing on alternative energy hardware will enable the utility to invest wisely in the future. (7)

Photovoltaic cells convert the sun's energy directly into electricity. Perhaps these little silicon rectangles or wafers may one day power electric knives, cordless drills, and innumerable other convenience appliances. The **solar calculator** is actually powered by nickel-cadmium batteries that are charged by the sun or artificial light. Three-quarters of one hour of summertime sunlight will provide ten hours of calculator time. This calculator has been used hundreds of hours but has never been purposely charged. (8)

The automobile accounts for 55 percent of all energy consumption in California. Yet, when given a choice of items that might be sacrificed in the name of energy reduction, few people would choose the automobile. Unless one lives in a city with adequate public transportation, one is by necessity a victim of automania—even though 54 percent of all automobile trips involve a distance of less than 8 kilometers (5 miles). Rather than give up the auto altogether, wouldn't it be better to opt for a vehicle that would consume less energy, wouldn't pollute, and would still get you where you wanted to go? The smog-free, silent Elektrikar that Rod Kaylor developed is one solution.

While Rod was in the Navy, he suffered an allergic reaction to organic solvents, and it took him fifteen years to outgrow the problem. The allergy was so intense that he had to have someone get gas for his car. For this personal reason, and because electric vehicles are much more practical in urban settings, Rod began to research the electric passenger car.

Rod Kaylor's **Elektrikar** has a powerful 30-horsepower DC continuous-duty shunt motor (100 horsepower peak) set into a low-weight 840-kilogram (1850-pound) fiberglass body. Low body weight provides good acceleration and radial tires on magnesium wheels reduce rolling resistance. Furthermore, the body of the car is engineered for aerodynamic soundness, which increases range. The heart of the auto is a 72-volt 220-ampere-per-hour lead-acid battery that, if properly nurtured, will provide a 640-kilometer (400-mile) range for as little as $1 worth of electricity. If zip is important, the four-speed transmission can withstand a speed of up to 112 kilometers per hour (70 miles per hour), although range will be substantially reduced.

Much of the research concerning electric transportation modes is devoted to storage batteries. The old "diehard" just can't take the frequent charge-discharge that it would be subjected to in an electric car. Batteries must be deep-cycle and extra-heavy-duty to withstand the physical beating. When electric transportation becomes the order of the day, batteries will have to be standardized. At present, battery research is variable: there's our old standard lead-acid, the zinc system—and Ford and GM are working on sodium-sulfur and lithium-chloride batteries, respectively. It's obvious that the battery must be standardized when you consider the local battery station will replace the gas station.

What role will the electric vehicle play in future transportation decisions? Rod Kaylor believes that the majority of our transportation modes—autos, buses, trams, subways, and whatever else may be invented—will be electrically powered. This will come to pass for three reasons: (1) there are just too many people to make it practical for everyone to own a car, especially in urban areas; (2) air pollution created by the internal combustion engine is causing a problem so grave that local municipalities may themselves restrict traffic; (3) fossil fuels will be in such short supply, or so expensive, that gasoline (and other fuels) will make the private ownership of automobiles almost impossible. Oil should be used to manufacture materials such as plastic insulation, food products, and other building materials, instead.

Electric passenger vehicles make sense from another angle. Gasoline will probably reach $1 per gallon in 1977. We are spending $80 million a day on imported oil, which is affecting our balance of payments. Finally, 90 percent of all automobile trips are under 32 kilometers (20 miles), in cars whose engines operate at about 37 percent efficiency at such distances. On all fronts—economy, energy, and ecology—electric vehicles are sound transportation alternatives. (9)

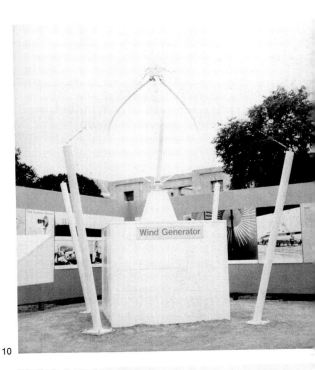

Wind Generator

Bicentennial Conservation Technology. In 1976, the red carpet was rolled out in Washington, D.C., in honor of this nation's 200th birthday. As part of the celebration, the Energy Research and Development Administration (ERDA), the Federal Energy Administration (FEA), and the Department of Housing and Urban Development (HUD) presented an exhibit of the latest developments in the solar-energy industry and related fields. Among the many attractions were a Darrius Wind Turbine (an electric wind generator) and a photovoltaic apparatus in which sunlight is converted into electric energy. The sun-energized solar cells are able to slowly turn a platform holding a large reflecting sculpture (these solar cells are similar to those used to power the solar calculator). The technology for converting the sun's energy into electricity was developed during aerospace experiments. The costs for a photovoltaic apparatus are prohibitive for the average consumer, but an economical device is currently being researched. 10

One significant development that was not on display but described in literature was a Litek energy-saving lightbulb. The bulb uses about 30 percent of the electrical energy that an incandescent bulb would require, and it fits standard fixtures. The projected operational cost of the Litek bulb over its 20,000-hour operating lifetime is $30.80 which is low compared to the $83 that it would cost to operate the 26 100-watt incandescent bulbs it would replace (conventional bulb life is only about 750 hours). About 20 percent of the electrical energy consumed in the United States goes for lighting, 11 percent of which is incandescent. Nationwide use of this new electrodeless fluorescent bulb would reduce the fuel required for lighting by up to 500,000 barrels a day.

Though the exhibit in Washington was not as visually impressive as some architecturally designed solar homes, the government should be commended for its efforts in alerting the public to alternative-energy applications. (10/11) 11

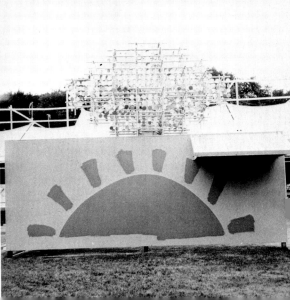

Conclusion

The information presented in the preceding pages is but the tip of the iceberg: these alternatives are only a smattering of what exists today. And like the glacier from which that iceberg was born, the potential for alternative energy use and conservation is vast. With our technological know-how and huge energy appetite, we have the incentive to solve the immediate international energy crisis.

The facts indicate that our energy appetite is indeed insatiable. In a 1972 study Stanford Research Institute designated over one hundred separate uses for energy in four broad categories: residential, commercial, industrial, and transportation. Focusing only on space- and water-heating energy use, the study indicated that 23.5 percent of all energy consumed in the United States went for these purposes.[1] Energy for space heating is second only to energy used for transportation. As we have attempted to show, space- and water-heating readily lend themselves to solar applications, so it's shocking that huge quantities of scarce fossil fuels are still being consumed for these purposes.

Private industries place a great deal of pressure on politicians (and on each other) to insure the protection and expansion of vested interests—many of which are wasteful energy-consumptive activities. For example, in 1968 electric toothbrushes accounted for 800 million kilowatt-hours of energy use. At an average rate of four cents per kilowatt-hour, that is $3,200,200 worth of energy. More important, this rather frivolous use of energy is something we can no longer afford. Unfortunately, people have been led to believe that these are necessary conveniences for maintaining our standard of living, and besides, they don't use much energy. On the contrary, in 1968 "necessary" appliances like garbage disposals, electric knives, toothbrushes, and blankets consumed over 4.5 billion kilowatt-hours of energy.[2] A reassessment of energy-use priorities must not be put off too long.

The United States, with 6 percent of the world's population, is leading the way in consumption of energy. In the last 150 years this country has consumed two trillion barrels of oil that the earth's bowels took three billion years to create. There is a lot of conflicting information about energy reserves, but the point is that money can be withdrawn from the bank for so long be-fore it runs out. At current rates of use, world fossil fuel reserves will probably be exhausted in about seventy-five years.[3] Far in advance of that 2050 date we will undoubtedly suffer blackouts, fuel rationing, and other inconveniences.

The average person would probably be more receptive to the use of solar, wind, and other energies if the federal government were conducting a more vigorous promotional campaign. Actually, the government is more committed to alternative energy, especially solar, than most people realize. From fiscal 1974 to 1977 the Energy Research and Development Administration's solar budget increased from $7.6 million to $286.8 million, and in August 1975 ERDA foresaw as much as 25 percent of the nation's energy coming from solar technologies by the year 2020.[4] ERDA's concerns, however, are being directed toward mass production of commercialized units that would be cost competitive. As a result, much of the budget is being spent on high-technology wind generators, photovoltaics, solar thermal power, ocean thermal power, and bioconversion of solar energy into organic matter. All these approaches are necessary, but they tend to discourage regional development and subsume local energy needs under national solutions. In other words, the government is going to solve the energy problem in cooperation with big business, irrespective of individual needs.

The federal government clearly intends to develop alternative energies, but it sees these as long-range applications that will follow nuclear energy, the development of America's outer continental shelf oil, and increased coal mining. According to Frank Zarb, former Federal Energy Administrator, these last three will be sufficient for the foreseeable future.[5] On the contrary, these are only Band-Aid measures for a large wound, for like all other finite energy sources, these fuels are limited. In addition, all—particularly nuclear energy—are so polluting and detrimental to the environment that it is immoral to consider them as more than minor transitional uses on our way to real energy independence. The sun is the ultimate nonpolluting energy source that will meet our needs in a healthy way.

What is the optimistic outlook for living with, rather than without, energy? Of number-one priority is conservation. Only a few ideas have been highlighted here.

A Twin Rivers, New Jersey, study of residential-use energy brings into focus some of the more subtle energy losses we incur.[6] Errors of only one-half degree Fahrenheit in thermostats can cause a loss of 4–5 percent in fuels consumed in winter; the same would occur during the summer with air conditioning. Home heating systems are so inefficient that only about one-half of the heat generated by natural-gas heaters ever reaches the intended area in single-story dwellings. The figures are even worse for multistory structures. The point is that zonal modes would reduce energy consumption by about 25 percent. Pilot lights consume 42 percent of all the energy used in gas stoves and 9 percent in gas furnaces. Electric-spark starters would almost completely eliminate this ridiculous waste. If you looked around your own home, you could probably find many more things that could be done to conserve energy. Conservation consciousness means that you spend the few extra dollars to caulk, seal, insulate, shutter, adjust, and clean your own living space so that you will consume less energy. A home retrofit program of this nature will cost about $400 and pay for itself in three to five years, depending on where you live.

The National Mineral Wool Association has estimated that if we use good insulation techniques in 75 percent of the new homes built, upgrade insulation in 25 percent of existing structures, and install storm windows on 12 percent of older homes, we would shave $3.1 billion from our energy bill by 1982. In ten years the nation could enjoy a $17.1 billion cumulative saving at a cost of only $6.4 billion to consumers.[7]

The so-called alternative energies like solar and wind were the energies prior to the advent of the fossil-fuel epoch. But because the almighty dollar was almost everyone's god, these renewable resources fell from favor for a temporary affair with inexpensive fossil fuels. As these fuels have become more expensive, interest in the alternatives has revived, but people still hesitate to commit themselves to using power from the wind and sun because they believe it is not yet economically feasible. They fail to realize two points: one, many energy alternatives are already cost competitive and cost effective; two, no amount of money can purchase something that doesn't exist, and it is only a matter of time before fossil fuels will be depleted.

A second priority is what I call passive technology. Basically this means a way of siting, designing, and building in a fashion that will complement the immediate environment. Your life and your needs should be integrated into the natural surroundings so that they have a minimal effect on nature. Whether an existing house is being retrofitted (remodeled) or a new house is being built, the intent should be passive if possible— that is, conserving without consuming energy.

When Charles and I started on this project we knew that there had to be better solutions to our energy concerns than the nuclear or coal alternatives. Little did we realize that the answer to our needs was shining in the sun and blowing in the wind. After being in over thirty solar houses and seeing hundreds of ways to conserve and use appropriate technology, ambivalent speculation on the potential of alternative energy is frustrating to us. Speculation is necessary only to determine which one of the alternative energy approaches is best for your micro-climatic situation.

It may be utopian to think that Americans will rise up and reshape their consumption patterns. But daily, through education and example, that's exactly what is happening. New ideas, new energies, new leadership, are exposing the fallacies embodied in the overconsumptive, environmentally degrading corporate industrial state. The people discussed here are catalysts: they should inspire each of us to look at our ecosystem in a manner that will heal existing wounds. More importantly, our value judgments must be flexible and far reaching, so that whatever we choose for ourselves will insure continued opportunities for our children.

[1] Stanford Research Institute, "Patterns of Energy Consumption in the U.S. Executive Office of the President," January 1972.

[2] Ibid.

[3] U.S. News and World Report, "We Should Have Started Yesterday," October 4, 1976.

[4] Science, "Solar Energy Reconsidered: ERDA Sees Bright Future," August 15, 1975, pages 538–39.

[5] Frank Zarb, "Nuclear Energy: The Time for Decision," speech before Commonwealth Club of California, July 11, 1975.

[6] Newsweek, "Snugging up for Winter," October 10, 1976.

[7] Smithsonian, "Houses Designed with Nature: Their Future Is at Hand," December 1975.

Alternative Energy Vocabulary

ABSORBER PLATE Portion of flat plate collector that absorbs sun's energy.

AC Alternating current, the "conventional" public utilities current.

ACTIVE SYSTEM A solar system requiring pumps or fans to move fluids, a mechanical system.

AQUACULTURE Fresh-water fish farming.

BANCO A sitting, lying, or lounging area made of adobe.

BATCH DIGESTOR A methane digestor that is filled, decomposes, and is subsequently emptied and re-filled.

BEADWALL A Steve Baer invention whereby tiny styrene beads are blown between two panes of glass for insulation and removed for direct-gain heating.

BERM A man-made mound or small hill of earth, in this case next to the wall of a building.

BIO-GAS See *Methane.*

BTU (British Thermal Unit) A heat-energy unit that will raise one pound of water one degree Fahrenheit (English system).

CALORIE A heat-energy unit that will raise one gram of water one degree Centigrade or Celsius (metric system).

CELLULOSE FIBER An insulation material made from recycled newspaper and having about same insulation value as fiberglass.

CLERESTORY or CLEARSTORY The wall of a room that goes above the adjoining roof and is pierced with windows.

CLIVUS MULTRUM A waterless composting toilet.

COLLECTOR PANEL A device insulated on three sides and open to the sun for heat absorbtion on the fourth side.

COOLTH The quality or state of being cool in temperature.

CONCENTRATING COLLECTOR A collector panel that is curved to concentrate the light or heat to a small area or point.

CONDUCTION Heat transfer directly through a material.

CONTINUOUS FLOW Either a methane or water-heating system where the material circulates continuously through the system.

CONVECTION Heat transfer created by the motion of air or water resulting from a difference in temperature (density) and the action of gravity.

DARRIUS A vertical axis eggbeater type of wind turbine used to generate electricity.

DC Direct current, the current from batteries and wind electric generators.

DEGREE DAY (Based on English system) An indication of how severe (cold) the weather is, based on a temperature of 65° F. If the average ambient outdoor temperature was 50° F. for the day, there would be fifteen degree days for that twenty-four hour period.

DORMER A projection on a sloping roof that forms a vertical wall suitable for windows or other openings.

ENERGY CYCLE A Rodale invention that uses pedal power to perform a number of household and gardening chores.

FAN COIL A heating device whereby air is forced by a fan across pipes or tubes containing a hot fluid.

FILON Brand name for a fiberglass material used to cover collectors, greenhouses, etc.

FIN TUBE A collector plate made up of tubes attached to sheet of metal or sheets of metal.

FLAT-PLATE COLLECTOR (See *Collector Panel*) Always flat.

GREENHOUSE EFFECT The physical phenomenon whereby light waves are admitted through a transparent structure but long-wave radiation is restricted from being reradiated to the atmosphere.

GRAY WATER Waste water from washing activities that does not contain excrement.

GLAZING The material used as collector covering that is almost transparent to short-wave solar radiation.

HEAT EXCHANGER A device used to transfer heat from fluid on one side of a barrier to fluid on the other.

HEAT LAG The time it takes for a heated material to reradiate absorbed heat.

HEAT PUMP An electric heating/cooling unit that absorbs heat from a low-temperature source (like air or water) and either delivers it as heat or coolth (in a refrigeration cycle) to a space. Produces more heat energy units than electrical energy units consumed.

HEAT SINK An area in a structure that absorbs and stores heat either from direct or transported solar radiation.

HOLISTIC Organic or functional relationship between parts and wholes.

INTEGRATED SYSTEM A tying together of all the facets of biotic (living) and abiotic (nonliving) parts in a community.

KALWALL Brand name of a fiberglass material used to cover collectors, greenhouses, etc.

KINETIC INSULATION Movable insulation, i.e. insulated shutters or insulated swimming-pool covers.

LONG-WAVE RADIATION Heat waves emitted from heated material like water or concrete.

METHANE A gas produced from anaerobic decomposition of organic material comprised of about 70 percent methane and 30 percent carbon dioxide, actually bio-gas.

MYLAR Brand name of a fiberglass material used to cover collectors, greenhouses, etc.

NET ENERGY The total amount of energy necessary to produce a product, i.e. from the energy used to manufacture the equipment to mine the fossil fuel, to the transportation of that finished fossil-fuel product to the retail outlet.

NEXTAL A very black coating that readily absorbs the sun's heat.

OFF-PEAK POWER Energy, usually electrical, used at a time when demand for the energy is low (7 A.M.–8 A.M. and 5 P.M.–7 P.M. are times of peak-power demand).

PASSIVE SYSTEM A system employing siting and orienting, selected building materials, and landscaping to take advantage of solar energy, and consuming no additional energy once installed.

PHOTOVOLTAIC Silicon cells capable of converting solar energy directly into electricity.

PLENUM A duct that, when heated, acts to initiate the movement of air.

RADIATION The process of giving off energy in the form of waves.

RETROFIT To remodel in an energy-conscious fashion using passive and/or active solar applications.

R FACTOR The resistance against loss of heat from a warm area to a cooler area imported by any material or still air.

ROCK STORAGE A mass of rocks in which heat may be stored—a heat sink.

ROLL BOND A kind of absorber plate of either copper or aluminum in which narrow channels have been embedded.

SAVONIUS A vertical-axis S-shaped rotor used for generating either mechanical or electrical energy as a result of wind.

SOLAR BATTERY A confined area that is capable of absorbing and storing heat for use when there is no sun, generally a glass-enclosed area with a water heat sink.

STACK OR CHIMNEY EFFECT The movement and stratification of warm and cold air—warm air always rises to the highest point.

SYNERGISTIC The combined effects of all the parts of a community or system working together.

THERMAL MASS A warm body, in this case an inanimate material like adobe, concrete, or water.

THERMISTORS An electrical resistor made of a material whose resistance varies according to the temperature.

THERMOGRATE A C-shaped fireplace grate that draws cool air in at the bottom portion of a tube and emits fire-warmed air at the top of the tube.

THERMOPANE Double- or triple-pane windows.

TROMBE WALL A massive wall covered with glass and vented at top and bottom to allow for air circulation.

VAPOR BARRIER A construction device impervious to the passage of moisture or air.

VIGAS Logs cut in the forest, skinned, and used as beams.

WATER GRATE A fireplace grate that allows water to pass through so the water can be heated.

Where to Go for Hardware and Further Information

In the United States

SOLAR GREENHOUSES

Helion, Box 4301, Sylmar, Ca., 91342, Attn: Elliott Freeman.

Mark Scanlon, 645 Lake Mary Rd., Flagstaff, Ariz. 86001. Ariz. Solar Eng. Assn., Solar Greenhouse Operations.

Bill Yanda, Director, Solar Sustenance Project, Route 1, Box 107AA, Santa Fe, N.M. 87501 (505) 445-7550.

Jerry Lahr, Hydro-Container Culture Systems, 2664 55th St., San Diego, Ca. 92104 (714) 262-6059. (Solar hydroponics.)

Joe Ennis, Poplar Branch, North Carolina 27965. (Methane and greenhouses.)

HARDWARE AND SOFTWARE

Dearing Solar Energy Systems, 12324 Ventura Blvd., Studio City, Ca. 91604. (Swimming-pool cover.)

Catel Manufacturing, Inc., 235 West Maple tura Blvd., Studio City, Ca. 91604. (Swimming-pool insulation.)

Solar Squares, The Pool Cover Company, 514A 17th St., Huntington Beach, Ca. 92648.

Heliotrope Gen., 3731 Kenora Dr., Spring Valley, Ca. 92077. (Differential thermostat in house.)

Sun Power Systems, Inc., 1121 Lewis Ave., Sarasota, Fla. 33577. (Minto wheel—solar heat engine.)

Kalwall Corporation, 1111 Candia Rd., P.O. Box 237, Manchester, N.H. 03105. (Collector glazing and solar products.)

Wisper Cool, Triangle Engineering Co., P.O. Drawer 38271, Houston, Texas 77088. (Wind-powered roof ventilator.)

Custom Solar Products Co., 4468 Industrial St., Simi Valley, Ca. 93063 (805) 527-2535. (Solar heaters, heat exchangers, solar panels.)

Division of Building and Community Systems, Office of Conservation, ERDA, Washington, D.C. 20545. (LITEK energy-efficient light bulb.)

Reflect-O-Screen, Inc., 7521 E. Second St., Scottsdale, Ariz. 85251.

Duro Test Corporation, 2321 Kennedy Blvd., North Bergen, N.J. 07047. (Energy-efficient lighting systems.)

Edmund Scientific Co., 605 Edscorp Bldg., Barrington, N.J. 08007. (Numerous books and materials on alternative energy.)

John C. Bowen, Power Systems Group, Ametec Inc., Hatfield, Pa. 19440. (Selective coatings.)

Enthone, Inc., Box 1900, New Haven, Conn. 06508. (Selective black coating.)

Rho Sigma, Inc., 15150 Raymer St., Van Nuys, Ca. 91405. (Solar controls, sensors, pumps, and instrumentation for solar systems.)

Zurn Industries, Inc., 5533 Perry Hwy., Erie, Pa. 16509. (Mini-dishwasher.)

Bristol Fiberlite Industries, 3200 S. Halladay St., Santa Ana, Ca. 92705 (714) 540-8950. (Skylights.)

Killer Watt Corporation, 2638 Yates Ave., Los Angeles, Ca. 90040. (Energy-saving lighting systems.)

EDUCATIONAL INSTITUTIONS

George Mansfield, Department of Mechanical Engineering, San Diego State Univ., San Diego, Ca. 92115.

Bob Plumb, Physics Department, Chico State College, Chico, Ca. 95926. (Influence of fog on solar reception.)

Brent Porter, School of Architecture, Pratt Institute, Brooklyn, N.Y. 11205.

Malcolm Lillywhite, Domestic Technology Institute, P.O. Box 2043, Evergreen, Colo. 80439.

University of Minnesota, School of Architecture, 110 Architecture Bldg., Minneapolis, Minn. 55455. Attn: Dennis Holloway.

Goddard College, Plainfield, Vt. 05667 (802) 454-8311. Dan Chodorkoff, Jim Nolfi, Murray Bookchin.

Chico State University, Chico, Ca. 95926 (916) 895-6116. Raleigh Burger (916) 354-7718 (home). (Retrofit on corner of Second and Hazel. Solar Energy Retrofit Project.)

Don Aitken, Environmental Sciences Department, San Jose State University, San Jose, Ca. 95100.

Dr. J. Taylor Beard, University of Virginia, Charlottesville, Va. 22903. (Solar testing of Solaris equipment in Blue Ridge Mountains.)

Lee Johnson, Editor, *Rain* magazine.

Rain, A Directory of Environmental Information Research in Pacific Northwest, 2270 N.W. Irving, Portland, Or. 97210.

The Center for Environmental Research, School of Architecture and Applied Arts, University of Oregon, Eugene, Or. 97403. Attn. Steve Baker/John Reynolds.

Southern California Institute of Architecture, 1800 Berkeley St., Santa Monica, Ca. 90404 (213) 829-3482.

Massachusetts Institute of Technology, Lincoln Laboratory, Lexington, Mass. 02173.

Wright-Ingraham Institute, 1228 Terrace Rd., Colorado Springs, Colo. 80904. Attn: Kathryn Toben.

Alvin Converse, Thayer School of Engineering, Dartmouth College, Hanover, N.H. 03755.

University of Arkansas, Department of Agricultural Engineering, 101 Agricultural Engineering Building, Fayetteville, Ark. 72701 (501) 575-2351. Attn: Thomas Rokeby. (Solar poultry brooder house.)

California Polytechnic State University at San Luis Obispo, San Luis Obispo, Ca. 93401. School of Architecture & Design, Professor Haggard. (Analyzed skytherm house of Harold Hay.)

Arizona State University, Tempe, Ariz. 85281, Architectural Foundation. John I. Yellott or Jeffery Cook.

Colorado State University, Fort Collins, Colo. 80521, Solar Energy Applications Laboratory, Fort Collins, Colo. 80523.

George Washington University, Wash., D.C. 20006, Prof. Ali Kiper. (Monitoring a Thomason systematized house.)

Ohio State University, Columbus, Ohio 43210. Mechanical Eng. Dept., 206 W. 18 Ave., Columbus, Ohio 43210. Prof. Charles Sepsy. (Solar heated house.)

State University at New Paltz, New Paltz, N.Y. 12561. Jerome Kerner, Coordinator of Environmental studies.

Santa Clara Solar Research Institute, 275 N Fourth Street, San Jose, Ca. 95112.

CONSTRUCTION

Mike Corbett, 244 Diablo, Davis, Ca. 95616 (916) 756-5941. Developer/contractor—Village Homes.

Storek & Storek, Richard Storek & Glen Storek, 149 9th St., San Francisco, Ca. 94100. (Lite dwell system for Sierra Club.)

Robert Terossi, Terossi Construction Co., Quechee Lakes, Vermont 05059.

Acorn Structures, John Bemis, Dept. CSM6, Box 250, Concord, Mass. 01742. (Free solar-heating bulletin and solar house information.)

COLLECTOR PANELS

Olin Brass, East Alton, Ill. 62024. (Roll-bond collector plates.)

Sky-Therm Process, Inc., 945 Wilshire Blvd., Los Angeles, Ca. 90017. (Passive water collectors.)

Sunworks, 669 Boston Post Rd., Guilford, Conn. 06437. (Solar collectors and literature.)

Alten Corporation, 2594 Leghorn St., Mountain View, Ca. 94043. (Do-it-yourself water-heating systems and insulation.)

Garden Way Laboratories, c/o Douglas Taff, P.O. Box 66, Charlotte, Vt. 05455. (Collector panels, solar water-heater, and do-it-yourself-plans.)

Burke Rubber Co., 2250 S. 10th St., San Jose, Ca. 95112 (408) 297-3500. Dennis Tankersley. (Solar swimming-pool heaters.)

Tranter Steel, 735 East Hazel St., Lansing, Mich. 48909. (Econocoil absorber plate.)

Caster, Terrance R., Pres., (714) 440-4646, Energy Systems, Inc., 634 Crest Dr., El Cajon, Ca. 92021 (714) 447-1000. (Copper tube aluminum fin panel.)

Bay Area Solar Collectors, 3068 Scott Blvd., Santa Clara, Ca. 95050 (408) 985-2272. Derek Douglas.

Amatec, John C. Bowen, Mgr., Power Systems, 1 Spring Ave., Hatfield, Penna. 19440 (215) 822-2971. (Manufactures panels being used by Santa Clara Recreation Center.)

Larry Anderson, Technical Director Engineering Program, c/o Lockheed, 3251 Hanover St., Palo Alto, Ca. 94304 (415) 493-4411, ext. 45904. (Panels for Santa Clara Recreation Center—Panels made by Amatec.)

Solartec Corporation, 8250 Vickers St., San Diego, Ca. 92111 (714) 560-8434. (Sun-tracker solar collectors, etc.)

Sunstream, Grumman Houston Corp., P.O. Box 365, Bethpage, N.Y. 11714. (Collectors with convex glazing, like those on Energy House.)

Falbel Energy Systems Corp., 472 Westover Rd., Stamford, Conn. 06902. Gerald Falbel, Pres. (Pyramidal Optics Solar House.)

Fafco Inc., 138 Jefferson Drive, Menlo Park, Ca. 94025. (Low-cost collectors for swimming pool and domestic hot-water heating.)

Raypack, Inc., 31111 Agoura Rd., P.O. Box 5790, Westlake Village, Ca. 91359. (Domestic hot-water systems.)

Solergy, Inc., Ron Smith, Pres., 150 Green St., San Francisco, Ca. 94111. (High heat, nested, extruded aluminum collector.)

Copper Development Assn., Inc., 405 Lexington Ave., New York, N.Y. 10017. (Copper solar collector industries list and other copper products.)

Solar Energy Products, Inc., 1208 N.W. 8th Ave., Gainesville, Fla. 32601 (904) 377-6527.

Sun Water Co., 1112 Pioneer Way, El Cajon, Ca. 92020.

Solar Applications, Inc., 7926 Convoy Court, San Diego, Ca. 92111 (714) 292-1857.

Solar Energy Dept., Revere Copper & Brass, Inc., P.O. Box 151 Rome, N.Y. 13440.

WASTE TREATMENT AND METHANE

Minuse Systems, Inc., 206 No. Main, Suite 300, Jackson, Ca. 95642. (Waste treatment.)

Fred Varani, Bio-gas of Colorado, Inc., 5620

Kendall Ct., Unit G, Arvado, Colo. 80002. (Methane.)

P.E.E. WEE, Inc., P.O. Box 108, Grass Valley, Ca. 95945. Jim Phillipson, Gene Elliott. (Waterless toilet.)

Recreational Ecology Conservation of U.S., Inc., 9800 West Bluemound Rd., Milwaukee, Wisc. 53226. (Self-contained water conserving toilet.)

Clivus Multrum, 14A Eliot St., Cambridge, Mass. 02138. (Composting toilet.)

Envirovac, 701 Lawton Ave., Beloit, Wisc. 53511. (Vacuum waste-treatment systems—uses air instead of water.)

Domestic Environmental Alternatives, P.O. Box 92, Hathaway Pines, Ca. 95233. Mike Skinfield, Tom Scheller.

ARCHITECTURE

Zoe Works, Garth Collier, 70 Zoe St., San Francisco, Ca. 94107.

Quigley Architecture, 662 State St., San Diego, Ca. 92101. Rob Quigley, Environmental Architect.

Lee Butler (Architect in San Francisco), 3375 Clay St., San Francisco, Ca. (415) 563-9531.

Interactive Resources, 39 Washington Ave., Pt. Richmond, Ca. 94801 (415) 236-7435. Thomas Butt.

John and Lori Hammond, Living Systems, Rt. 1, Box 170, Winters, Ca. 95694 (916) 753-3033.

Alten Associates, Suite 200-D, 3080 Alcott, Santa Clara, Ca. 95051 (408) 247-6967. Frank Verprauskus 225-7946 (home), or Barry Scott.

Richard Crowther, 310 Steele St., Denver, Colo. 80206 (303) 355-2301 or 388-1875. Crowther Solar Group.

David Wright, 960 Camino Santander, Santa Fe, N.M. 87501 (707) 785-2397, or Sea Ranch, Ca. 95497.

Blue Minges, Blue Sun Limited, Farmington, Conn. 06032. Architect.

Malcolm Wells, Box 183, Cherry Hills, N.J. 08002.

Roy Mason, Box 558, Arlington, Va. 22216. Designer and contractor of urethane foam and solar homes.

CONSULTATION—DESIGN—IDEA PEOPLE

Hewlett Packard Co., Palo Alto, Ca. 94300, Martin McFee. (Solar heating at company as well as retrofitted local homes.)

Norman Saunders, 15 Ellis Rd., Weston, Mass. 02193 (617) 894-4748. Professional engineer.

Earth Dynamics, Inc., Box 1175, Boulder, Colo. 80302 (303) 447-8168. Design Group.

R.H. Bushnell, 502 Ord Drive, Boulder, Colo. 80303 (303) 449-7421. Professional engineer.

Travis L. Price, 519 East 11th Ave., N.Y., N.Y. 10009. Designer.

Dr. Geo. Lof, Solaron Corp., 4850 Olive St., Denver, Colo.

Zomeworks Corp., Steve Baer, P.O. Box 717, Albuquerque, N.M. 87103. Solar design.

Wormser Scientific Corp., c/o Eric Wormser, 88 Foxwood Rd., Stamford, Conn. 06903. Solar design.

Sennergetics, 18621 Parthenia St., Northridge, Ca. 91324. Solar system design and sales.

H.E. Thomason, 6802 Walker Mill Rd., S.E., Wash., D.C. 20027 (301) 336-0009, 336-4042, 336-5329. Solar design and hardware.

Bruce Corson, Office of State Architecture, P.O. Box 1079, 1500 5th St., Sacramento, Ca. 95805 (916) 445-4711 (General Services), or 445-8432 (office). Solar design.

Douglas R. Coonley, Box 49, Harrisville, N.H. 03450 (603) 827-3086. Design, research, and consulting.

Bruce Wilcox, Berkeley Solar Group, 1815 Francisco St., Berkeley, Ca. 94703 (415) 843-7600. Consultation.

Jack Schultz, Schultz Field Enterprises, Inc., Solar Utilities Co., San Diego, California.

Jersey Devils, 56 Buttonwood St., New Hope, Pa. 18938. Steve Badanes. Design for solar-home applications.

Dimetrodon Corp., Rt. 1, P.O. Box 160, Warren, Vt. 05674. Bill Maclay. Cluster of ten solar-heated houses.

Dave Springer, Natural Heating Systems, 207 Cortez Ave., Davis, Ca. 95616 (916) 756-4558. Consultation.

Paul Shippee, Colorado Sunworks, P.O. Box 455, Boulder, Colo. 80302, or 1945 Grove St. (in back). Solar systems/consultation.

Ken Herrington, 769 22nd St., Oakland, Ca. 94612. Water heating fireplace and solar wares.

Dave Rozell, San Jose State University, Department of Environmental Studies Bldg. University of San Jose, California. 95192. Consultation.

Mike Jantzen, Box 172, Carlyle, Ill. 62231. Solar design.

Ted Bakewell, 8820 Ladue Rd., St. Louis, Mo. 63124 (314) 862-5555 (work), or (314) 427-6163 (home). Design and consultation.

Richard Merrill, 24 Glen Dr., Scotts Valley, Ca. 95066. Energy Primer co-editor, methane and alternative agriculture, Radical Agriculture editor.

Wilson Clark, Hidden Valley Ranch, Rt. 2, Box 111, Cle Elum, Wa. 98922. Energy for Survival, author.

WIND POWER

Dwyer Instruments, Inc., P.O. Box 373, Junction Ind. 212 & U.S. 12, Michigan City, Indiana 46360. Wind-speed instruments.

Meteorology Research, Inc., Box 637, Altadena, Ca. 91001. Meteorology equipment.

Kahl Scientific Instrument Corporation, P.O. Box 1166, El Cajon, Ca. 92022. Meteorological instruments.

U.S.D.A.-A.R.S., Louis Liljedahl, Rural Remote Areas Wind Energy Research, Bldg. 303, Agricultural Research Center—East, Beltsville, Md. 20705. Grants for wind-energy applications.

Windworks, Box 329, Rt. 3, Mukwanngo, Wisc. 53149. Retrofitted generator, do-it-yourself-plans.

Dempster Industries, Inc., P.O. Box 848, Beatrice, Nebr. 68310. Water-pumping windmill.

Earthmind, Mariposa, Ca. 95338 (209) 966-5255. Mike Hackleman, Mark Dankoff, Vanessa Naumann. Retrofitted wind generators and other energy applications plus numerous publications.

Upright Scaffolds, 1013 Pardee St., Berkeley, Ca. 94701. Wally Johnson, Pres. Manufacturing a 4000-watt tri-bladed wind turbine. (Wind Power System design.)

Sencenbaugh Wind Electric, 2235 Old Middlefield Way, Mtn. View, Ca., or P.O. Box 11174, Palo Alto, Ca. 94306 (415) 964-1593. Small-size U.S. built wind generator and monitoring equipment.

Real Gas & Electric, Soloman and Denise Kegan, Rich Polack, P.O. Box "A", Guerneville, Ca. 95446. Wind and other alternative energy systems.

Windy-Ten Ltd., 150 Orchard View, P.O. Box 111, Shelby, Mich. 49455. Attn: Jack Maas. Dutch-type windmills.

Wind Power Systems, Inc., 8871 Balboa, Suite A, San Diego, Ca. 92123, (714) 560-9452, Edmund L. Salter, Pres. Consultation and design for wind systems.

Aero Power, Tom Conlon, 432 Natoma, San Francisco, Ca. 94103. U.S.-built wind generator.

Charlie Hall, 50 Brook St., Barre, Vt. 05641.

Retrofitted wind generators of all kinds.

Dyna Technology, P.O. Box 3263, Sioux City, Iowa 51102. Wind charger, wind generators.

Aeromotor Water Systems, Braden Industries, Inc., Broken Bow, Oklahoma 74012. Water-pumping windmills.

Aero Power, Warren, Vt. 05674 Don Meyer. Wind generators and systems.

INTEGRATED SYSTEMS

New Alchemy Institute, Box 432, Woods Hole, Mass. 02543. John and Nancy Todd, Bill McLarney, Ty Cashman.

Max's Pot, Center for Maximum Potential Bldg. Systems, 6438 Bee Caves Rd., Austin, Texas 78746.

Farallones Institute, 15290 Coleman Valley Rd., Occidental, Ca. 95465. David Katz.

Cerro Gordo Community Assn., 704 Whiteaker St., Cottage Grove, Ore. 97424. (Page 190 EP.)

Brace Research Institute, MacDonald College of McGill University, Ste. Anne De Bellevue 800, Quebec, Canada (514) 457-6580, McGill University (514) 392-4311. Ron Alward, Paul Lawand.

Ecotope Group, 747 16 E., Seattle, Wa. 98112.

Organic Gardening and Farming, Organic Park, 22 Main St., Emmaus, Pa. 18049 (215) 967-5171.

Integral Urban House, Farallones Institute, 1516 5th St., Berkeley, Ca. 94710. Helga and Bill Olkowski.

GOVERNMENT AND PUBLIC UTILITIES

National Solar Heating and Cooling Information Center, P.O. Box 1607, Rockville, Md. 20850 (800) 523-2929.

Chuck Lischer, Dir., San Diego Gas Solar Collector program, Corner of 10th and Imperial, San Diego, Ca. 92101. This organization has two solar houses.

Southern California Gas Co., Rich Nemec, Public Relations, Project SAGE, Los Angeles, Ca. 90051 (714) 581-6123. Group of thirty-two apartment buildings retrofitted with solar hot-water systems.

City of Santa Clara, Santa Clara, Ca. 95054.

Pennsylvania Power & Light Co., 2 North Ninth St., Allentown, Pa. 18101. Solar-heated house.

Four Corners Regional Commission, U.S. Dept. of Commerce, Room 1898C, Wash., D.C. 20230. Regional funding commission for greenhouse and methane projects.

National Agriculture Research Center, Dr. Paul Thompson, Project Mgr., USDA—Agriculture Research Service, Beltsville, Md. 20705 (301) 344-2213. Solar dairy project.

NASA, Langley Research Center, Hampton, Va. 23665 (804) 827-3281. Attn: Joel K. Zoeffel. "Home of Future," open to public.

Solar Energy Industries Assoc., Suite 632, 1001 Conn. Ave., NW, Wash., D.C. 20036. Publishes directory of solar industry: promotes commercial advancement of solar energy. Membership.

ERDA—Technical Information Center, P.O. Box 62, Oak Ridge, Tenn. 37830. Publications on energy.

Pacific Gas & Electric, Energy Conservation and Services Dept., 77 Beale St., San Francisco, Ca. 94106.

Washington Natural Gas, 815 Mercer St., Seattle, Wa. 98111 (206) 622-6767.

Portland General Electric, 621 SW Alder, Portland, Or. 97223.

Department of Energy, 528 Cottage St. N.E., Salem, Or. 97310. Family Energy Watch Calendar.

ORGANIZATIONS

The Community Soap Factory, Esther Siegel/ Jeffery Woodside, 3156–18th St. NW, Wash., D.C. 20010. Formerly Community Technology, an organization working on self-reliance within the city.

Community Action Center for Appropriate Technology, Richard Saul, Room 500-A, Community Services Administration, 1200 19th St. NW, B-Bldg., Wash., D.C. 20506.

Citizens for Conservation & Solar Development, c/o George Lark, P.O. Box 49173, Los Angeles, Ca. 90049. Report on solar heating plans for greenhouses.

Southern Calif. Solar Energy Assn., City Administration Bldg., 202 C Street, San Diego, Ca. 92101.

Ecology Action/Common Ground, 2225 El Camino Real, Palo Alto, Ca. 94306 (415) 382-6752.

Northern California Solar Energy Assn., Robert Paterson, P.O. Box 1627, Richmond, Ca. 94802. Dues: $5.00/yr.

Volunteers in Technical Assistance, 3706 Rhode Island Ave., Mt. Rainier, Md. 20822. Attn: Laurel Durben. H_2O, wind.

Total Environmental Action, Box 47, Harrisville, N.H. 03450. Bruce Anderson. Design, publications, and workshops.

Intermediate Technical Development, Ltd. 9 King St., London, WC2 8HN, England. E.F. Schumacher's appropriate technology group.

New England Solar Energy Assoc., P.O. Box 21, Townshend, Vt. 05353. Newsletter, monthly meetings, membership.

New Mexico Solar Energy Assoc., c/o Architects, P.O. Box 1884, Taos, N.M. 87571. Publications & membership.

Alternate Consumer Energy Society, 4800 Oak Grove Drive, Pasadena, Ca. 91103. Access to alternate energy sources, including low-cost hardwares, technical assistance, and education. Associated with Jet Propulsion Lab.

Alternate Energy Systems, 150 Sandwich St., Plymouth, Mass. 02360. New England distributor for Rho Sigma, Fafco, and various woodheating and wind-power units.

PUBLICATIONS

SUN Catalog, Solar Usage Now, Inc., Box 306, Bascom, Ohio 44809. Solar Products Catalog—$2.00.

Wind Power Digest, 54468 C.R. 31, Bristol, Ind. 46507. $6.00/yr. for four issues.

A-Z Solar Products, 200 E. 26th St., Minneapolis, Minn. 55404. Solar Products Catalog. Fifty cents.

EARS—Environmental Action Reprint Service, 2239 East Colfax, Denver, Colo. 80206. Catalog of alternative energy publications.

Adobe News, Inc., P.O. Box 702, Los Lunas, N.M. 87031. $8.00/yr.—has much on solar adobe.

SOLAR AGE, Solar Vision, Inc., 260 East Main St., Port Jervis, N.Y. 12771. $20.00/yr. Excellent articles on what people are doing.

SPECTRUM, Alternative Sources of Energy, Rt. 2, Box 90A, Milaca, Minn. 56353. Alternative-technology equipment directory.

"Buying Solar," Mr. Joseph Dawson, Director of Public Affairs, Office of Consumer Affairs, Dept. of Health, Education, and Welfare, North Bldg., 330 Independence Ave. SW, Rm. 3310, Wash., D.C. 20201 (202) 245-6975.

AERO—Alternative Energy Resources Organization, 435 Stapleton Bldg., Billings, Montana 59101. $10.00/yr. for membership and newsletter.

Electric Vehicle News, P.O. Box 533, Westport, Conn. 06880. $10/yr.

Not Man Apart, Friends of the Earth, Commercial St., San Francisco, Ca. 94111. Environmental newsletter with much information on nuclear power industry and energy conservation (excellent up-to-date source of political activity). $20.00/yr.

Manager, Publications Marketing, The American Institute of Architects, 1735 New York Ave., NW, Wash., D.C. 20006. Hundreds of publications on architecture; many on energy conserving approaches.

Energy Reporter, Federal Energy Administration Citizen Newsletter, Federal Energy Administration, Wash., D.C. 20461.

Solar Energy Digest, P.O. Box 17776, San Diego, Ca. 92117. William Edmondson, Ed. $28.50/yr.—on top of latest happenings.

COUNTRYSIDE, Highway 19 East, Waterloo, Wisc. 53594. Small-scale farming and livestock journal.

Undercurrents, 11 Shadewell, Uley, Dursley, Gloucestershire, England. $7.50/yr.

RAIN Magazine, 2270 N.W. Irving, Portland, Or. 97210. Lee Johnson, Editor.

SOLAR ENGINEERING, Solar Engineering Publishers, Inc., 8435 N. Stemmons Freeway, Suite 880, Dallas, Texas 75247.

Mother Earth News, P.O. Box 70, Hendersonville, N.C. 28739. $10/yr.—all kinds of alternatives and ideas in life-style and hardware applications.

WATER POWER AND CONSERVATION

Bill Delp, Independent Power Developers, Inc., P.O. Box 1467, Noxon, Montana 59853. $2.00 for information packet.

Ecological Water Products, P.O. Box 509, Dunkirk, New York 14048. Water-conserving shower and faucet heads.

Noland Company, National Accounts Dept., 2700 Warwick Blvd., Newport News, Va. 23607. Flow control devices—water savers.

Grundfos Pumps Corporation, 2555 Clovis Ave., Clovis, Ca. 93612. Low-energy pumps.

The Whole Mother Earth Water Works (H_2O), c/o Edward Barberie, P.O. Box 104, Green Springs, West Va. 26722.

Department of Water Resources, P.O. Box 388, Sacramento, Ca. 95802. Water conservaton information on home landscaping and water-conserving devices.

Water Control Products/NA, Inc., 1100 Owendale, Suite E, Troy, Mich. 48084 (313) 689-1700.

Moody Sprinkler Co., 3020 Pullman St., Costa Mesa, Ca. 92627 (714) 556-8730.

WOOD POWER

Thermograte, 51 Iona Lane, St. Paul, Minn. 55117. Fireplace grate to make fireplace more efficient (also Sears).

"Old Country" Appliances, P.O. Box 330, Vacaville, Ca. 95688. Sole U.S. importer of Tirolia (Austria) coal- and wood-burning ranges.

Torrid Manufacturing Co. Inc., 1248 Poplar Pl. SO., Seattle, Wa. 98144. Torrid air—forced-air recycling unit installed in flu pipe of wood stove/heater.

Vermont Castings, Inc., Box 126, Prince St., Randolph, Vermont 05060. Defiant Parlor Stove —excellent American-made heater.

Blazing Showers, P.O. Box 327, Point Arena, Ca. 95468. Stove-pipe water heater.

Champion Home Builders Co., Solar Furnace, 5573 E. North St., Dryden, Mich. 48428.

Wells Fireplace Furnaces, P.O. Box 7546, 1750 W. Ajo Way, Tucson, Ariz, 85713. Bill Wells (602) 294-4648. Energy-efficient fireplace.

Portland Stove Foundry Co., Portland, Maine 04104. Wood stoves and heaters.

The Atlanta Stove Works, Inc., P.O. Box 5254, Atlanta, Georgia 30307. Franklin stoves.

Ashley Automatic Heater Co., 1604 17th Ave. SW, P.O. Box 730, Sheffield, Alabama 35660. Stoves and heaters.

TRANSPORTATION

Electric Passenger Cars, Inc., P.O. Box 17700, San Diego, Ca. 92117. Electric cars.

Electric Vehicle Council, 90 Park Ave., New York, N.Y. 10016.

Kaylor Energy Products, 1918 Menalto Ave., Menlo Park, Ca. 94205. Electric car.

In Canada

CENTERS OF INFORMATION

Energy Probe, 43 Queen's Park Crescent East, Toronto, Ontario (416) 978-7014. (Good information library and source of contacts.)

Pollution Probe Ottawa, 53 Queen Street, Suite 54, Ottawa, Ontario K1P 5C5 (613) 231-2742. (Environmental group active in energy issues; a number of publications available through them.)

Ontario Science Centre, 770 Don Mills Road, Toronto, Ontario (416) 429-4100. (The Science Centre has working models of many renewable energy harnessing technologies.)

Institute of Man and Resources, P.O. Box 2008, Charlottetown, P.E.I. C1N 4M1. (Good source of information on solar heating and other renewable energy systems.)

Solar Energy Society of Canada Inc. (SESCI). Head office: P.O. Box 1353, Winnipeg, Man., R3C 2Z1. Membership: $10.00 per year. (The national organization has affiliated local chapters equipped to supply specific information, publications, or contacts. The chapters also hold regular meetings.) SESCI—B.C.: Richard Kabulski, 1271 Howe Street, Vancouver, B.C. V6Z 1R3. SESCI—Alberta: Jerry Wright, 2009 Avord Arms, 10020-103 Avenue, Edmonton, Alta. T5J 0G8. SESCI—Saskatchewan: Peter Catania, University of Regina, Regina, Sask., S4S 0A2. SESCI—Saskatoon: Robert Dumont, Department of Mechanical Engineering, University of Saskatchewan, Saskatoon, Sask. S7N 0W0. SESCI—Manitoba: Gren Yuill, 1666 Dublin Ave., Winnipeg, Man. R3H 0H1. SESCI—Thunder Bay: Sharon McFadden, Physics Department, Lakehead University, Thunder Bay, Ontario. SESCI—Sarnia: W. Himmelman, 1034 Lombardi Dr., Sarnia, Ont., N7S 2E2. SESCI—London: Jim Bolton, Department of Chemistry, University of Western Ontario, London, Ontario. SESCI—Toronto: Dan Shatil, P.O. Box 396, Station D, Toronto, Ont., M6P 3J9. SESCI—Kingston: M. J. Wolstencroft, 385 Maple Ridge, Kingston, Ontario, K7N 5P1. SESCI—Ottawa: Jim McAuley, Public Information Branch, N.R.C., Montreal Road, Ottawa, Ontario K1A 0R6. SESCI—New Brunswick: Verne Ireton, 177 Kelly's Court, R.R.3, Fredericton, N.B.

An excellent list of goods, services, and information, prepared by Robert Argue, is the "Catalogue of Solar Heating Products and Services in Canada," Research Report No. 12 (February 1977), available from the Office of Energy Conservation/Renewable Energy, Resources Branch, Dept. of Energy, Mines, & Resources, 17th floor, 580 Booth Street, Ottawa, Ontario K1A OEA.

Bibliography and Sources

Alternate Celebrations Catalogue, 3rd ed., Alternatives 1975, Greensboro, North Carolina.

Alward, Ron. "Solar Steam Cooker." Brace Research Institute, St. Anne de Bellevue 800, Quebec, Canada. October 1972.

"An Interview with David Wright." *Adobe News,* Issue 9 and 10. Los Lunas, New Mexico, Adobe News Inc., 1976.

America's Energy Crisis. *Newsweek,* January 1976.

Baer, Steve. *Sunspots,* Albuquerque, New Mexico, Zomeworks Corp., 1975.

Bainbridge, David. "Jon Hammond: Another Quiet Solar Energy Pioneer." *Mother Earth News,* No. 36, November 1975: 120–125.

Baron, Winnie. "A Visit with Karen Terry." *Adobe News,* Issue 10, Los Lunas, New Mexico, Adobe News Inc., 1976.

Behrman, Daniel. *Solar Energy, the Awakening Science.* Little, Brown and Co., Boston, 1976.

Birkhead, Gene et al., ed. Running Creek Field Station Report. Wright Ingraham Institute, April 1976.

Bortz, Brenda. "New Crops for America?" *Organic Gardening and Farming,* July 1975.

Botwright, Ken. "Flush Toilet Soon May Be Antique." *Boston Globe,* August 12, 1974.

Branch, Diana. "Cycling Toward Energy Efficiency." *Organic Gardening and Farming,* May 1976.

Bregg, Gary N. et al. "God Bless Mr. Savonius." *Mother Earth News,* No. 36, November 1975: 129.

"Building Ideas," *Better Homes & Gardens.* Des Moines, Iowa, Special Interest Publications, Spring 1976.

Calrulles, Janet. "Growing Things." *Canyon Courier,* Evergreen, Colorado, July. 29, 1976: 7, 18.

Carroll, Rick. "The Bay Area Men Who Get a Charge Out of Electric Cars." *San Francisco Chronicle,* September 10, 1976, p. 12.

Cervinka, Vashek et al. "Energy Requirements for Agriculture in California." Department of Food and Agriculture, and University of California, Davis, January 1974.

Chalon, Mark, and Wilson, Quentin. "The Sun Dwelling Demonstration Center." *Adobe News,* Issue 10, Lcs Lunas, New Mexico, Adobe News Inc., 1976.

Clark, Wilson. *Energy For Survival.* Garden City, New York, Anchor Press/Doubleday, 1975.

Clark, Wilson. "Energy for Survival." Lectures at Goddard College, Summer 1975.

Clews, Henry. "Electric Power from the Wind." Solar World, P.O. Box 7, East Holden, Maine, 1974.

Clegg, Peter. *New Low-Cost Sources of Energy for the Home.* Charlotte, Vermont, Garden Way Publishing, 1975.

Commoner, Barry. *The Poverty of Power.* Alfred Knopf, New York, 1976.

Concern, Inc., Eco-Tips #5. Energy Conservation, Washington, D.C. 1973.

Congressional Quarterly. *Continuing Energy Crisis in America.* CQ, Inc., Washington, D.C., 1975.

Coonley, Douglas R. "An Introduction to the Use of Wind." Total Environmental Action, Church Hill, Harrisville, New Hampshire, July 1975.

Crawford, Berry. "The Energy Crisis: A Blessing in Disguise." *The Futurist,* August 1976.

Crowther, Richard L. *Sun Earth.* 1976, p. vii, The A.B. Hirschfield Press Inc., Denver, Colorado.

Daniels, Farrington. "Direct Use of the Sun's Energy." New York, Ballantine Books, 1974.

Daniels, Richard. "On the Energy Scene Old Sol Is the Star." *San Diego Union,* San Diego, California, May 16, 1976.

DeKorne, James B. "An Experimental Aquaculture System." *Mother Earth News,* No. 31, January 1975:76–78.

DeKorne, James B. "The Solar Heated Greenhouse." *Mother Earth News,* No. 36, November 1975:101–104.

DeKorne, James B. *The Survival Greenhouse.* The Walden Foundation, New Mexico, 1975.

Demperwolff, Richard F. "Sunpower: The Heat's On for Real," *Popular Science,* September 1975:63–65, 119.

Department of Economics, "Solar Distillation," United Nations, New York, 1970.

Diamond, Stuart. "Wastage Ups Energy Use by 50% in Nation." *Modesto Bee,* November 26, 1976.

Eccli, Eugene. *Low Cost Energy Efficient Shelter for the Owner & Builder.* Pennsylvania, Rodale Press Inc., 1976.

Elder, Leon. "Plug Your Tub into the Sun." *Hot Tubs,* Vintage Books, May 1975, p. 57.

Energy and the Built Environment: A Gap in Current Strategies, American Institute of Architects, May 1974.

"Energy Task Force." 519 E. 11th St. N.Y.C., N.Y., Unity Press, 1975.

Ennis, Joe. "A Greenhouse Food Supply Project." *Green Revolution.*

"Environmental Effects of Energy Use." *The Science Teacher,* December 1972.

ERDA, A National Plan for Energy Research, Development and Demonstration: Creating Energy Choices for the Future. Superintendent of Documents, June 28, 1975.

Faltermayer, Edmund. "Solar Energy Is Here, But It's Not Yet Utopia," *Fortune,* February 1976.

Friggins, Paul. "What You Should Know About Solar Heating." *Readers Digest,* July 1976.

Fry, John L., and Merrill, Richard. "Methane Digestors for Fuel, Gas and Fertilizer." Newsletter #3, Santa Barbara, California, New Alchemy Institute, Spring 1973.

"Garden Ideas & Outdoor Living." *Better Homes & Gardens,* Des Moines, Iowa, Special Interest Publications, 1976.

Gelles, Teresa. "Family Builds Solar Home, Discovers It's Beautiful." *Menlo-Atherton Recorder,* Menlo Park, California, April 28, 1976:3.

Green, Terrance. "San Diegans Take Lead in Solar Field." *Los Angeles Times,* March 28, 1976.

Green, Terrance. "Blossoming Solar Energy Field Marked by Contrasts." *Los Angeles Times,* April 4, 1976.

Green, Terrance. "Solar Energy Industry Focus Two Major Problems." *Los Angeles Times,* April 18, 1976.

Greene, Wade. "The New Alchemists." *New York Times Magazine,* August 8, 1976.

Hackleman, Michael. Newsletter #1A, Supplement to *Wind & Wind Spinner,* Boyer Rd., Mariposa, California, July 1975.

Hackleman, Michael. "Earthmind Newsletter Two, Wind & Solar Energy." Boyer Rd., Mariposa, California, July 1976.

Hackleman, Michael. *The Homebuilt, Wind-Generated Electricity Handbook.* Culver City, California, Peace Press, 1976.

Hackleman, Michael. *Wind and Wind Spinners.* Culver City, California, Peace Press, 1976.

Hamer, John. "Solar Energy: Where We're At." *Modesto Bee,* November 21, 1976.

Hammond, Allen. "Solar Energy Reconsidered: ERDA Sees Bright Future." *Science,* August 15, 1975.

Hammond, Jonathan et al. *A Strategy for Energy Conservation.* Energy Conservation Ordinance Project Prepared for the City of Davis. Davis, California, 1974.

Hammond, Jonathan. "Proposal For: An Energy Conservation Service." Living Systems, Rt. 1, Box 170, Winters, California, December 1975.

Hayden, M.B., and Thompson, P.D. "Solar Thermal Energy Application in the Milking Parlor." USDA, APS, Beltsville, Maryland, 1976.

Headley and Springer. "A Natural Connection Solar Crop Drier." University of West Indies, St. Augustine, Trinidad.

"A Heat Pump for the House," Changing Times, *The Kiplinger Magazine,* January 1976:16.

Herrington, Ken. Solar Water Heaters, Herrington-Olson Photography, Oakland, California.

"How to Make a Solar Cabinet Drier for Agricultural Produce." Brace Research Institute, MacDonald College of McGill University, March 1973.

"How to Make a Solar Still." Brace Research Institute, Ste. Anne de Bellevue 800, Quebec, Canada, February 1973.

"How to Build a Solar Water Heater." Brace Research Institute, Ste. Anne de Bellevue 800, Quebec, Canada, February 1973.

Ingraham, Elizabeth Wright. "Lead Time for As- sessing Use: A Case Study." *Science,* Octo- ber 1976, pp. 17–22.

Kelbaugh, Douglas. "Kelbaugh House." A paper by Douglas Kelbaugh.

Kennedy, Edward. Lecture on "The Energy Crisis" at Commonwealth Club of California, January 31, 1975.

Kern, Ken. *The Owner Built Home.* Charles Scribner's Sons, New York, 1975.

Leckie, Jim et al. *Other Homes and Garbage.* Sierra Club Books, 1975.

Lesley, Jason. "Sun Power Here." *Salisbury Evening Post,* November 7, 1975, p. B1.

Love, Sam. "Houses Designed with Nature: Their Future Is at Hand." *Smithsonian,* De- cember 1975.

Love, Sam. Lecture at Goddard College week of July 15, 1975.

Mason, Roy. "Architecture Beyond 2000." *The Futurist,* Vol. IX, No. 5, October 1975:235– 246.

Mazria, Edward, and Winitsky, David. *Solar Guide and Calculator.* The Center for Envi- ronmental Research School of Architecture and Applied Arts, University of Oregon, Eu- gene, Oregon, September 1976.

McNabrey, Jim. "Coming: New Ways to Power Your Farm." *The Furrow.*

Merrill, Richard, ed. *Radical Agriculture.* Harper Colophon, New York, 1976.

Moran, Edward. "Larry J. Romesberg Cooks with Bio-Gas." *Popular Science,* December, 1975:95,109.

Moran, Edward. "Five Solar Water Heaters You Can Build." *Popular Science,* May 1976:99– 103.

The Mother Earth News, No. 32. "The Plowboy Interview," p. 6; "The Patch-Whitely Methane Plant," p. 86; Special Windplant Section, p. 99.

The Mother Earth News, No. 35. "The Plowboy Interview," Peter van Dresser, p. 8.

A Nation of Energy Building by 1990, American Institute of Architects.

"The New Organic Gardening." Experimental Farm, Pennsylvania, Rodale Press Inc.

"New Prototype Tested." *Wind Power Digest,* No. 4, Spring 1976.

Omer, Henry. "$7.00 a Year Heats the House." *Popular Mechanics,* February 1965, pp. 89– 93.

Parson, Robert A. "Windmills Are Not the An- swer." *California Rancher,* August 1975.

Pimentel, David et.al. "Food Production and the Energy Crisis." *Science,* Vol. 182, November 2, 1973, pp. 443–449.

"Planning Guide for the Garden Way." Sal-R- Tech Solar Heat Collector System, Charlotte, Vermont, Garden Way Laboratories, 1975.

Energy Primer. Portola Institute, Fremont, Cali- fornia, Recke-Parks Press, Inc., 1974.

"Revival of the Family Farm." *The Modesto Bee,* November 26, 1976, p. A2.

Reynolds, Jule. "The Integral Urban House." *The Mother Earth News,* No. 42, November 1976:125–129.

Roberts, Rex. *Your Engineered House.* New York, N.Y., M. Evans and Co., Inc., 1964.

Rockwell, Susanne. "The Homes that Jonathan Builds." *The Winters Express,* Winters, Cali- fornia, May 6, 1976.

Rowe, Ken. "That Lazy Old Sun Put to Work in Portola Valley." *Palo Alto Times,* May 3, 1976:3.

"Saving Energy on the Farm." *California Rancher,* April 1975, pp. 10–12.

Schumacher, E.F. *Small Is Beautiful.* Harper & Row, New York, 1973.

Scientific American, ed., *Energy and Power,* Freeman and Co., San Francisco, California, 1971.

"Self-Reliance—The Key to the Small Farm Future." *Countryside,* August 1976, p. 10.

Shelter. Bolinas, California, Shelter Publica- tions, 1973.

Sheudan, Norman R. "Solar Heating a Swim- ming Pool." Solar Research Notes No. 6, University of Queensland, Department of Mechanical Engineering, 1975.

Shurcliff, W.A. *Solar Heated Buildings, A Brief Survey.* 11th ed., 19 Appleton St., Cambridge, Massachusetts, November 11, 1975.

Shurcliff, W.A. *Informal Directory of the Or- ganizations and People Involved in the Solar Heating of Buildings.* 19 Appleton St., Cam- bridge, Massachusetts, December 12, 1975.

Skurka, Norma. "The Solar Way: Passive." *New York Times Magazine,* November 30, 1975.

Smyser, Steve. "Methane from Manure at the Organic Demonstration." *Organic Gardening and Farming,* October 1974.

Smyser, Steve. "In Pursuit of Zero-Discharge Household." *Organic Gardening and Farm- ing,* May 1976.

"Solar." *Sunset,* November 1976:79–89.

"The Solar Furnace." *Home Building and Re- modeling.*

"Solar Heat Collector for Drying Fruits & Vegetables." *Sunset,* August 1976.

"Solar Power for Your Home—How Practical Now?" *Changing Times,* March 1976, pp. 43–46.

Stanford Research Institute. *Patterns of Energy Consumption in the U.S.* Executive Office of the President, January 1972.

Stepler, Richard. "Solar Water Heaters." *Popu- lar Science,* May 1976:104–105.

Stepler, Richard. "Solar Architecture." *Popu- lar Science,* July 1976:48–52, 96.

Terry, Karen. "Karen Terry's House." *Solar Age,* November 1976.

Thomason, Harry E. *Solar Homes & Solar House Models,* 2nd edition. Edmund Scientific Co., 1972.

Thomason, Harry E. and Harry J. Solar House Plans II-A, Edmund Scientific Co., 1975.

Thome, Joe. "Windmills—Clean Power Genera- tion Could Be a Breeze." *Modesto Bee,* December 29, 1974.

Thompson, P.D. "Solar Energy for Milking, Par- lor Heating & Cooking." USDA, APS, Belts- ville, Maryland, 1975.

Thompson, P.D. "Some Rules of Thumb for Solar Energy Application to Dairying." USDA, APS, Beltsville, Maryland.

Tobias, Andrew. "Solar Energy Now: Why Aren't We Using It More?" *New West,* June 7, 1976, pp. 32–39.

Todd, Nancy J., ed. *The Journal of the New Al- chemists,* No. 3, Woods Hole, Massachusetts, New Alchemy Institute Inc., 1976.

Todd, Nancy J., ed. *The Journal of the New Al- chemists,* No. 2, New Alchemy Institute Inc., 1974.

"Vacation House Warmed by Sun Power." *House and Garden,* 1976.

Van Der Ryn, Sim et al. Farallones Institute Newsletter, January 1976.

van Dresser, Peter. *A Landscape for Humans.* Albuquerque, New Mexico, Biotechnic Press, 1973.

van Dresser, Peter. "Ghost Ranch." *Solar Age,* November 1976.

Wells, Malcolm B. "The Architects Are Killing Us." *Building Official & Code Administrator,* July 1972.

"The Whirlwind Comforts the Skeptics." *Time,* January 21, 1974, p. 22.

Wilhden, John. "Solar Energy, The Ultimate Powerhouse." *National Geographic,* March 1976, pp. 381–397.

Williams, Robert. "The Potential for Fuel Con- servation." Hearing on the California Nuclear Safeguards Initiative, December 2, 1975.

Woods, Chuck. "Reducing Fuel Costs with Solar Energy." University of Florida, Institute of Food & Agricultural Sciences, Research Report for Fall 1975.

Wright, David. "Adobe." *Solar Age,* July 1976.

Wright-Ingraham Institute, Newsletter 5, Fall 1975.

Yanda, Bill, and Rick Fisher. *The Food and Heat Producing Solar Greenhouse.* John Muir Press, 1977. $5.00.

Zarb, Frank. Lecture, "Nuclear Energy: The Time for Decision" at Commonwealth Club of California, July 11, 1975.

Zeman, Tom. "Solar Power Now." *Ramparts,* April 1975.

Zmuda, Joseph. "Solar Architecture, A Western Approach." *Popular Science,* July 1976:53.